CHILD ABUSE AND NEGLECT

The Guilford School Practitioner Series

EDITORS

STEPHEN N. ELLIOTT, PhD
University of Wisconsin–Madison

JOSEPH C. WITT, PhD
Louisiana State University, Baton Rouge

Recent Volumes

Child Abuse and Neglect: The School's Response
CONNIE BURROWS HORTON and TRACY K. CRUISE

Traumatic Brain Injury in Children and Adolescents: Assessment and Intervention
MARGARET SEMRUD-CLIKEMAN

Schools and Families: Creating Essential Connections for Learning
SANDRA L. CHRISTENSON and SUSAN M. SHERIDAN

Homework Success for Children with ADHD: A Family–School Intervention Program
THOMAS J. POWER, JAMES L. KARUSTIS, and DINA F. HABBOUSHE

Conducting School-Based Assessments of Child and Adolescent Behavior
EDWARD S. SHAPIRO and THOMAS R. KRATOCHWILL, *Editors*

Designing Preschool Interventions: A Practitioner's Guide
DAVID W. BARNETT, SUSAN H. BELL, and KAREN T. CAREY

Effective School Interventions
NATALIE RATHVON

DSM-IV Diagnosis in the Schools
ALVIN E. HOUSE

Medications for School-Age Children: Effects on Learning and Behavior
RONALD T. BROWN and MICHAEL G. SAWYER

Advanced Applications of Curriculum-Based Measurement
MARK R. SHINN, *Editor*

Brief Intervention for School Problems: Collaborating for Practical Solutions
JOHN J. MURPHY and BARRY L. DUNCAN

Academic Skills Problems: Direct Assessment and Intervention, Second Edition
EDWARD S. SHAPIRO

Social Problem Solving: Interventions in the Schools
MAURICE J. ELIAS and STEVEN E. TOBIAS

Instructional Consultation Teams: Collaborating for Change
SYLVIA A. ROSENFIELD and TODD A. GRAVOIS

Child Abuse and Neglect

THE SCHOOL'S RESPONSE

♦♦♦

Connie Burrows Horton
Tracy K. Cruise

♦

THE GUILFORD PRESS
New York   London

© 2001 The Guilford Press
A Division of Guilford Publications, Inc.
72 Spring Street, New York, NY 10012
www.guilford.com

Printed in the United States of America

This book is printed on acid-free paper.

Last digit is print number: 9 8 7 6 5 4 3 2

Library of Congress Cataloging-in-Publication Data

Horton, Connie Burrows.
  Child abuse and neglect : the school's response / Connie Burrows Horton, Tracy K.
Cruise.
      p.   cm. — (The Guilford school practitioner series)
  Includes bibliographical references and index.
  ISBN 1-57230-673-4 (hardcover)
  1. Child abuse—Prevention.   2. Child abuse—Reporting.   3. School social work.
I. Cruise, Tracy K.   II. Title.   III. Series.
  HV6626.5 .H67 2001
  372.17′8—dc21   2001023132

About the Authors

♦

Connie Burrows Horton, PhD, is a licensed clinical psychologist and a certified school psychologist, and currently is the Director of Counseling and Consultation Services at Illinois Wesleyan University. She earned her master's degree in counseling at California State University, Fullerton, and her PhD in educational psychology in the school psychology program at the University of Texas, Austin. Throughout her career, Dr. Horton has been involved in the field of child abuse through research, practice, and training roles in a variety of practice and academic settings.

Tracy K. Cruise, PhD, is an Assistant Professor of Psychology at Western Illinois University (WIU). She received her master's degree in clinical psychology and her PhD in school psychology from Illinois State University. She teaches and supervises child psychotherapy for both the school psychology and clinical/community mental health graduate programs at WIU. Her research and clinical experience focuses on the consequences and mediators of child maltreatment and how such experiences may affect the lives of individuals and families.

Preface

♦

Child maltreatment has finally been recognized as one of society's most insidious problems. Child abuse and neglect, previously "taboo" subjects, have received markedly increased public and professional attention in recent decades. Clinicians report treating scores of victimized, often traumatized, children and their families. Researchers confirm alarming incidence and prevalence rates, serious consequences, and widespread adverse risk factors. Specialized professional organizations and conventions have been established; focused journals have been developed; a rapidly growing literature has emerged. All of these efforts have increased the knowledge base and helped to inform the practice of psychologists, counselors, social workers, and other mental health professionals working in the field of child maltreatment.

Schools, too, have been asked to respond. By the 1980s schools were recognized as "the major social institution concerned with the development of children." Therefore, it was argued, they should "assume a major responsibility in facilitating, reporting, and participating in the delivery of services to the abused" (Volpe, 1980, p. 3). Given their extensive out-of-home contact with students, school professionals do have a unique opportunity to identify and respond to child maltreatment (Horton, 1995; James & Burch, 1999; O'Toole, Webster, O'Toole, & Lucal, 1999; Tite, 1994; Tharinger & Vevier, 1987). Additionally, because of their expertise in child development, family systems, assessment, counseling, and consultation, school psychologists and school counselors, in particular, have been called upon to be involved in the school's response to child abuse and neglect (James & Burch, 1999; Vevier & Tharinger, 1986). There is evidence that many have tried to accept the challenge and be more involved (Tharinger, Russian, & Robinson, 1989).

In recent years, however, concerns have shifted to youth violence and school violence in particular, as alarming stories of school shootings have repeatedly shocked the nation (Garbarino, 1999). Schools are being asked to respond to these crises, prevent future violent incidents, and identify those at risk for committing such horrific acts. Do schools still have time to be also concerned about child abuse and neglect, or are there now these more pressing issues? In fact, as documented in *Early Warning, Timely Response* (Dwyer, Osher, & Warger, 1998) and other studies on school violence, these are not separate matters. Instead, one of the most important steps that schools can take to prevent future violence is to identify and effectively respond to students who have been maltreated. Those who commit violent acts often are victims of severe abuse and neglect, or as Garbarino (1999) describes them in *Lost Boys: Why Our Sons Turn Violent and How We Can Save Them*, they are the "rejected and neglected, ashamed and depressed." Thus, now more than ever, there should be an urgency among school professionals regarding their need to respond to the critical issues of child abuse and neglect.

Although school personnel may be very concerned about these matters and may want to be responsive to children who have been abused and neglected, they may not know where to begin. Unfortunately, many have had limited exposure to the topic of child maltreatment in their university training. Self-directed continuing education is also a challenge. Resources directed specifically at school-based professionals are limited, and the more general abuse literature is growing so rapidly that keeping up to date is quite difficult.

Therefore, the purpose of this book is to integrate the findings from the recent abuse literature and apply them to school-based practice. Beyond statistics and conceptual ideas, we must always keep in mind that child maltreatment is a tragic phenomenon affecting the lives of *real* children. Thus, in addition to summarizing findings from the research literature, case illustrations are used throughout the text. The examples are hypothetical or are a compilation of details from several children. This approach allows us to "put a face" on the discussion, but still protect the privacy of the children and families we have worked with in our years of clinical experience in schools and other mental health settings.

Chapter 1 provides an overview of the field, definitions of maltreatment, and a review of the recent empirical literature regarding incidence and prevalence, risk factors, consequences, and mediators of child abuse and neglect. This sets the stage for the remainder of the book, which focuses on practical applications to school systems.

Chapter 2 addresses the critical topic of identifying child abuse and neglect—specifically, by being aware of potential indicators and by being prepared to respond effectively to students' disclosures. Once child abuse or neglect has been identified, reporting decisions must be made, so that is the focus of Chapter 3. The rationale and pragmatics of reporting are described, as are fears, systemic problems, and other obstacles to fulfilling the mandated role.

While these first chapters may be applicable to all educators, the remainder of the book emphasizes more clinical issues, of particular interest to school-based mental health practitioners. For example, the following two chapters address meeting the counseling and therapy needs of children who have been maltreated. Working with outside providers is discussed in Chapter 4, while school-based services are described in Chapter 5.

Chapter 6 addresses consulting with those in key positions in the life of a child who has been maltreated: teachers and parents. Suggestions for providing the needed information and support to those influential individuals are discussed and related resources are identified.

While other chapters address the response to maltreatment that has already occurred, Chapter 7 discusses the school's role in the ultimate goal, preventing child abuse. Components of effective programming and implementation pragmatics are reviewed.

Finally, Chapter 8 addresses the understandable response to working in the field of child maltreatment: compassion fatigue. Self-assessment and self-care methods are discussed in an effort to promote healthy, long-term involvement in this critical field.

This book is offered with the hope that school professionals find the material relevant and useful in their daily practice. As schools are increasingly asked to play a broader role in the lives of children, school personnel will need to stay well informed about child maltreatment and well prepared to prevent, detect, and respond to child abuse and neglect. This up-to-date synthesis of the literature with a specifically school-based focus is intended to facilitate these challenging roles.

For the children . . .

CONNIE BURROWS HORTON
TRACY K. CRUISE

Acknowledgments

♦

Without the support of many, this book would not be possible. We are grateful to so many of our professional colleagues, friends, and family members who supported us through this endeavor.

I, Connie, specifically would like to thank my ever-patient husband, Tim, and my precious children, Josh and Hannah, for enduring the focused time it took to complete this project. Additonally, I am grateful for the support I received from my siblings and my parents, John and Marilyn Burrows; for so many dear friends in my church family, especially the Kalmeses, Paynes, and Sharps, who sustained me; and for my special friends and colleagues in my peer supervision group, especially Tom and Cheri, and at Illinois State University, especially Jeff, Jayne, and Mark, who were an encouragement.

I, Tracy, am especially grateful to my husband, Jeff, for supporting and enduring this project and encouraging me when doubt was ever present and time was of the essence. I would also like to acknowledge the ongoing support from colleagues and staff at Western Illinois University, especially Jim Ackil and Paula Wise. The unwavering belief in and expectance of the completion of this book by my mother, Reba Schuder, and closest friend, Paula Dougherty, could not be more appreciated.

We both appreciate the assistance of the excellent reviewers and editors at The Guilford Press and our graduate assistants, who helped with various phases of the book along the way. We also want to recognize all of the school personnel who are on the "front lines" addressing child maltreatment issues on a daily basis. Finally, we are especially indebted to our previous clients and research participants who were courageous enough to share their experiences with us. They helped us to gain a very personal look at child maltreatment and its consequences.

Contents

♦

CHILD ABUSE AND NEGLECT

CHAPTER 1

♦♦♦

Overview of Child Maltreatment

♦

Child maltreatment has loomed as a serious social problem for centuries. Public recognition of the matter, however, is fairly recent. Dr. C. Henry Kempe, Dr. Brandt F. Steele, and colleagues drew the first significant attention to child abuse in the United States in their 1962 address to the American Academy of Pediatrics and publication in the *Journal of the American Medical Association* in which they coined the phrase "the battered child syndrome" (Kempe & Helfer, 1980). Concerns regarding children's health and welfare have continued to be at the forefront of social policy, professional practice, and public interest in the United States and throughout much of the world. National incidence rates consistently attest to the numerous children who are affected by maltreatment each year. For example, in 1997, over 3 million children in the United States were reported as possible victims of child maltreatment; nearly a million of those cases were *confirmed* victims of child abuse and neglect (U.S. Department of Health and Human Services [DHHS], 1999). Although these figures are high, retrospective studies of adults reflecting back on their childhoods reveal much higher prevalence rates. Reporting rates are clearly just the "tip of the iceberg."

Before examining incidence and prevalence rates further, definitions of child maltreatment should be addressed. The definitions found in the federal Child Abuse Prevention and Treatment Act (National Center on Child Abuse and Neglect [NCCAN], 1988) are used most commonly; however, many states have modified them, yielding no universally accepted legal definitions of child maltreatment. There are, however, ideological similarities across definitions. Thus, the following categories express broad conceptual explanations of five types of maltreatment: physical abuse, sexual abuse, emotional abuse, neglect, and witnessing domestic violence.

1

DEFINITIONS

Physical Abuse

Ms. Reed, Ben's teacher, escorted 7-year-old Ben and 9-year-old Kelly to the principal's office. The principal explained that a woman was coming to ask questions about their home life. When Mrs. Brown, the child protection caseworker, arrived, she told Ben and Kelly that Ms. Reed had been concerned about the frequent "accidents" Ben had been reporting to explain his bruises. Mrs. Brown said she would like to talk with them individually. The children huddled together like frightened animals, with Kelly constantly reassuring Ben that everything would be fine. Ben's eyes began to tear as Kelly tried to console him. Finally, Kelly agreed to leave Ben's side to talk to Mrs. Brown. Kelly told of multiple instances of being left in the care of her mother's boyfriend, who would hit Ben with whatever he could find—a belt, a clothes hanger, a Barbie, or even the leg from the coffee table that had broken Ben's fall when the boyfriend had shoved him across the room. Kelly sobbed as she told of her mother's believing the boyfriend's words that "it was an accident" rather than believing her and Ben. She also told of a recent occasion in which her mom "just stood there" while the boyfriend hit Ben in the face. Although Kelly's mom helped stop the bleeding, she reminded Ben that he should not have been "smarting off."

Physical abuse is an act of commission by a parent or caretaker characterized by the infliction of physical injury (English, 1998; Tower, 1992). Physical abuse of children may take many forms and vary in both severity and duration. Injuries from physical abuse may result from extended physical altercations (e.g., hitting, kicking, shaking) or brief, isolated incidents (e.g., being burned, thrown down stairs, bitten, poisoned). Physical abuse can be intentional, as some adults make a conscious decision to hurt a child. In some cases parents may intend to cause pain but not extensive injuries; in other cases the physical abuse may be the unintentional consequence of a parent's loss of self-control. Usually there is some recognition by caretakers of the wrongfulness of their actions and often an attempt to hide the abuse. Parents may tell the child what to say when asked about his/her injuries, threaten the child if he/she tells the truth, or try to cover the injuries with cosmetics or clothing, making it more difficult for educators to notice evidence of the abuse.

Physical abuse victimization appears to decline with age (American Association for Protecting Children [AAPC], 1985). The majority of physical abuse victims (65%) are under the age of 12, with a substantial percentage of these only 7 years old or younger (DHHS, 1999). Adolescents certainly are, at times, victims of physical abuse; however, very young children are more likely to suffer severe—even fatal—injuries (DHHS, 1999). Males and females seem to be equally at risk for physical abuse (52% and 48%, respectively; AAPC, 1988; DHHS, 1999); yet, boys are at greater risk for more severe physical abuse (AAPC, 1988).

The majority of perpetrators of physical abuse are parents (75%, DHHS, 1999). However, these figures may be inflated due to reporting definitions, which require *caretakers* to have committed the acts. There are no notable gender differences in rates of the parents perpetrating the abuse (DHHS, 1999).

Sexual Abuse

> When Mrs. Brown, the child protection caseworker, asked Kelly if her mother's boyfriend had ever harmed her, Kelly hugged her knees tightly to her chest and buried her head. After a long pause, she softly whispered that when the boyfriend smelled of beer that he would force her to touch his "thing." Kelly reported that on the one occasion that she refused, the boyfriend had beaten her brother, Ben, with the television remote and locked them both in their rooms until it was time for their mother to return from work.

Sexual abuse has been defined as "the involvement of dependent, developmentally immature children in sexual activities that they do not fully comprehend and therefore to which they are unable to give informed consent and/or which violate the taboos of society" (Krugman & Jones, 1987, p. 286). Although many think of sexual abuse as sexual contact between an adult and a child, the definition is much broader. Noncontact sexual acts (e.g., being forced to watch the perpetrator masturbate) may be involved, and the offender may be an adolescent or another child who has some power or control over the victim.

Sexual contact with children may include fondling of breasts and genitals, forced masturbation of themselves or the perpetrator, oral sex, digital penetration, or anal or vaginal intercourse. Noncontact abuse may include encounters with exhibitionists or voyeurs, solicitation to engage in sexual activity where no physical contact occurs, or exposure to, or involvement in, pornography (Courtois, 1993; Horton & Cruise, 1997a; Peters, Wyatt, & Finkelhor, 1986). Sexual abuse may involve a combination of these acts and will often progress from less to more invasive forms in an attempt to desensitize the child to sexual content or contact (Kaufman et al., 1998). For example, an offender may use sexual language around the child, expose himself to a child, then move to fondling, oral sex, and finally to intercourse (Courtois, 1993).

Definitions of sexual abuse, often based on age differences between the child and perpetrator, may suggest that most offenders are adults. However, empirical studies (Finkelhor & Dziuba-Leatherman, 1994; Kikuchi, 1995;

Ryan, 1997) in the past two decades illustrate that a significant portion of offenders are under the age of 18, with more recent findings indicating that prepubescent children also may molest other children (Cruise, 1999). Anecdotal reports by adult offenders indicate that many of them began offending as young as age 6 (Longo & Groth, 1983; Ryan, 1989).

In officially reported and substantiated cases, girls are about three times more likely than boys to experience sexual abuse (DHHS, 1999; NCCAN, 1988; Sedlack & Broadhurst, 1996). Retrospective studies of adults have also found an average of 2.5 females reporting a child sexual abuse experience for every male reporting victimization (Finkelhor & Baron, 1986). However, most acknowledge that the abuse of boys is still significantly underreported because boys are less likely to self-disclose abuse (Finkelhor & Baron, 1986).

Children are most vulnerable to sexual abuse between the ages of 3 and 15, with some studies noting particularly high rates between the ages of 8 and 12 (DHHS, 1999; Finkelhor & Baron, 1986; Sedlack & Broadhurst, 1996). In some cases, however, the abuse starts at much younger ages, even during infancy. Cases involving very young children are likely to be undercounted because the victim's rudimentary language skills and overall development prevent a credible disclosure. The average length of intrafamilial sexual abuse is 4 years, while extrafamilial abuse is generally much shorter in length, probably due to more limited access to the child victim (Courtois, 1993).

Males perpetrate the vast majority (80–95%) of sexual abuse, though there are certainly some cases in which female offenders victimize male or female children (Allen, 1991; Finkelhor, Hotaling, Lewis, & Smith, 1990). Female victims are more likely to be sexually abused by someone within their family (e.g., parent, stepparent, grandparent, uncle, cousin, sibling) (Courtois, 1993; Finkelhor, 1994; Larson, Terman, Gomby, Quinn, & Behrman, 1994). Males are more likely to be sexually abused by someone outside of the family. However, contrary to the myth that most perpetrators are strangers, even extrafamilial abusers are typically known by the child (e.g., neighbors, babysitters, friends of the family, coaches, teachers) (Finkelhor et al., 1990).

Offenders within and outside of the family may gain access to the child victim through deception or by direct approach through the use of psychological pressure, enticement, and encouragement. Children with family problems, poor supervision, and low self-esteem may be most vulnerable (Finkelhor, 1994), as offenders deliberately target children who are vulnerable and responsive to their attention. Thus, force is frequently not needed. There are cases in which force, threats, or use of strength are involved (Burgess & Groth, 1980), however, and adolescent offenders are most likely to engage these strategies (Kaufman et al., 1998).

Given the dynamics of sexual abuse, particularly the difference in power between the offender and the victim, a child victim will often keep the experience of sexual abuse a secret. Some children feel guilty. Others are deceived into thinking the experience is normal or educative. Children may believe the threats made to keep their silence or believe there are some "benefits" or "payments" for participating—or costs for refusing to do so.

The newest medium that offenders have begun using to reach vulnerable children is the Internet. A recent study surveying youths 10 to 17 years old found that 20% of those participants who regularly used (i.e., at least once a month) the Internet had received unwanted sexual solicitations and approaches during the past year (Finkelhor, Mitchell, & Wolak, 2000). In some instances, the solicitor attempted to gain further access to the minor via phone, mail, or in-person meetings. Parents and educators should remember that the Internet gives offenders easy access to many children. Children and adolescents who have poor boundaries, are emotionally needy, or are poorly supervised may be most vulnerable to their blandishments.

Emotional Abuse

The only attention Shauna ever received at home was when her mom would yell at her because the dishes were not done or the laundry not finished. Shauna was constantly reminded that she was "a mistake that never should have happened" and that she had ruined her mother's life. Shauna had come to believe her mother's statements that she was "dumb as a post" and would never do anything right. She knew this was the reason she never had the right answer when called on in class and why the other kids would never want to be her friend. Shauna sat alone and wondered why she even cared.

Emotional abuse includes treating a child in a way that is rejecting, degrading, terrorizing, isolating, corrupting, exploiting, or denying emotional responsiveness (e.g., love, care, support; Brassard & Gelardo, 1987) (see Table 1.1). Emotional abuse is the repeated acts and/or omissions of parents or caregivers in meeting the child's emotional needs and in helping to develop a positive sense of self and social competence (Garbarino, Guttman, & Seeley, 1986). The term "psychological maltreatment" is used by some to describe this form of abuse since it clearly has both cognitive and affective components. At the same time, this form of abuse relates to the core issues that are inherent in all forms of child maltreatment, and thus clarifies and unifies constructs (Brassard & Gelardo, 1987). That is, children who experience other forms of maltreatment, such as physical abuse, sexual abuse, or neglect, are also affected emotionally and psychologically. Still, emotional abuse can occur in isolation. It is possible for a parent never to be physically violent, never cross sexual boundaries, and continually provide adequate nutrition, education, and supervision, and still be emotionally abusive by making constant, degrading, hurtful comments. Although almost all parents have made

TABLE 1.1. Seven Behavioral Types of Emotional Abuse

Type	Description
Rejecting	Verbalizations or behaviors that communicate rejection or abandonment of the child, such as refusing to help a child or show affection
Degrading	Words or acts that belittle a child, such as insulting, name calling, or humiliating a child in public
Terrorizing	Verbalizations or actions that are meant to threaten or promote fear in a child, such as threats to the well-being of the child, a pet, or a loved one
Isolating	Actions by an adult that prevent the child from participating in normal social events or interactions, which may involve simple refusals or locking the child up
Corrupting	Encouragement or lack of redirection by the caregiver that reinforces antisocial behaviors, such as substance abuse, delinquent behavior, or aggression
Exploiting	Encouraging, permitting, or demanding a child to act in a way that will meet the needs of the caregiver or be to the caregiver's advantage
Denying emotional responsiveness	By ignoring or refusing to interact with the child, the caregiver deprives the child of necessary emotional (e.g., love, care, support) and physical stimulation

Note. Information for this table was obtained from the following sources: Brassard and Gelardo (1987); Garbarino, Guttman, and Seeley (1986); Miller-Perrin and Perrin (1999); and Tomison and Tucci (1997).

a derogatory comment to their child at least once, it is the repeated or chronic nature of these actions that makes them abusive.

Emotional abuse occurring alone may be more difficult to recognize, as it is more vague than other types of abuse. That is, it is difficult to know where to "draw the line" and say that a particular parental behavior is truly emotionally abusive rather than just poor parenting. Emotionally abusive parents may blame their children and may lack awareness of how their own actions are affecting their children negatively.

Victims of this type of maltreatment may also have a difficult time recognizing their experience as abuse and thus frequently do not report it to others. There may be no observable signs of what has happened to them. Yet, these parental actions have injured their children's self-esteem and self-concept. Emotional abuse can have such a powerful impact because young children normally interpret what their parents say and do as truth. Children cannot test parental behavior against reality to know that just because a parent says a child is stupid does not make it so (Morgan, 1994). Children come to believe they are the way their parent describes them or treats them (i.e., stupid, worthless, ugly), and they may even begin to act accordingly (Miller-Perrin & Perrin, 1999).

Emotional abuse, which appears to be evenly distributed across both age and gender, is one of the least common types of maltreatment reported and substantiated by child protective service (CPS) agencies (DHHS, 1998, 1999; NCCAN, 1988). This could be due in part to the variations in definitions, but it may also be largely due to individuals focusing on and reporting the more "obvious" co-occurring types of maltreatment. Thus, a concerted effort may not be made in reports to specify this type of abuse, even though it occurs simultaneously. When psychological maltreatment occurs in isolation, it is more nebulous, making it more difficult to identify, report, and substantiate. It is usually those extreme cases (e.g., locking a child in a closet for extended periods of time, threats of abandonment, or tying a child up) that are more readily reported, while more subtle instances (e.g., rejecting, ignoring, degrading, or permitting corrupting actions) go undetected and/or unreported.

Among children who are emotionally abused, the perpetrator is once again more often the parent. Both mothers and fathers equally emotionally abuse their children (DHHS, 1999). However, other caregivers (e.g., stepparents, babysitters, boyfriends/girlfriends) who psychologically maltreat children are more often men than women (males 80% to 90% vs. females 14% to 15%) (Sedlack & Broadhurst, 1996).

Neglect

Shelly sat crying by the fence on the middle school playground. She was alone and cold. The winter wind ripped through her torn windbreaker, and she felt chilled to the bone. Shelly knew that the other fourth graders did not like to play with her because she was not like them. They called her names like "Smelly Shelly" and "Salvation bin Shelly." Shelly did not have attractive clothes like the other children and felt lucky that the school provided her lunch because it was often the only meal she had all day. She spent most of her time at home and at school by herself. Her mother worked the second shift, and Shelly was left home to take care of her two younger brothers. She rarely had time to finish her homework and was failing most of her subjects, another reason she was not well liked. On the weekends Shelly's mom would be gone to her boyfriend's or he would be at their house with a few of his friends.

Neglect has been defined as "a form of maltreatment characterized by a chronic lack of care in the areas of health, cleanliness, diet, supervision, education or meeting of emotional needs, which places the child's normal development at risk" (Ethier, Palacio-Quintin, & Jourdan-Ionescu, 1992, p. 13). In defining child neglect, a reference is made to the standards of care believed necessary for the physical and psychological development of a child. Neglect occurs when those needs are not met at the minimal level required by the community and culture at that time, a situation that results in actual or potential harm (Dubowitz, Klockner, Starr, & Black, 1998; Garbarino & Collins, 1999).

National incidence studies undertaken by the National Center for Child Abuse and Neglect include three types of neglect: physical, emotional, and educational (see Table 1.2) (Sedlack & Broadhurst, 1996). The common dimension across these three types of neglect is the caregiver's failure to meet the needs of the child (Garbarino & Collins, 1999). This dynamic distinguishes child neglect from physical or sexual abuse, which involve the commission of an act by another that is harmful to the child. Child neglect, instead, involves omissions of appropriate parental activity. This makes operational definitions difficult. For example, at what age can a child be left unsupervised without it being neglectful? Defining the point at which a child slips from minimally satisfactory care to neglect is difficult (Helfer, 1987).

Although minimal standards of care are culture- and community-specific, research in the United States has shown some agreement across socioeconomic classes and some racial groups (e.g., African Americans, whites) as to conditions and situations that place a child at risk of harm (Dubowitz et al., 1998; Polansky & Williams, 1978). However, there is some disagreement among these groups as to which needs are most important (i.e., physical vs. psychological and emotional) (Dubowitz et al., 1998). Middle-income fami-

TABLE 1.2. Three Primary Subtypes of Child Neglect

Type	Definition
Physical neglect	Refusal or delay in seeking health or dental care; abandonment, expulsion of a child from the home, or the refusal of a runaway to return home; failure to meet nutrition, clothing, or hygiene needs; inadequate supervision, failure to provide an adequate and sanitary home, or failure to protect children from foreseeable hazards or dangers in and around the home
Emotional neglect	Inadequate attention to a child's needs for nurturance and affection; chronic or extreme exposure to domestic violence; permitting a child to use drugs, alcohol, or cigarettes; or refusal or delay of psychological care
Educational neglect	Permitted chronic truancy, failure to enroll a child in school, lack of supervision over the educational process, or inattention to specific educational needs (e.g., a learning disability)

Note. Information for this table was obtained from the following sources: Gelles (1999); Miller-Perrin and Perrin (1999); and Peterson and Urquiza (1993).

lies seemed to emphasize psychological needs more than physical needs, while lower-income families reported the opposite priorities (Dubowitz et al., 1998).

Additional factors that must be considered in determining neglect include the severity of a particular omission and whether the neglect is chronic or circumstantial (Ethier et al., 1992; Miller-Perrin & Perrin, 1999). Neglect is typically chronic, but even a single neglectful episode may have a highly detrimental outcome. For example, a young child left alone with matches, even once for only a few minutes, may well suffer horrific burns and thus become a victim of neglect. Most instances of neglect, however, result from chronic omissions by caregivers. For example, children who repeatedly come to school hungry, exhausted, in the same unwashed clothes, or without needed glasses or medications are the more typical cases of neglect.

Reasons for chronic neglect vary and may include an intellectual handicap, drug addiction, or emotional immaturity on the part of parents that results in a multiproblem family (Ethier et al., 1992). However, in some cases, an out-of-the-ordinary period of neglect may be the result of a recent stressor (e.g., a divorce, a parent's illness, or mental health concerns) that may be altering the parents' normal level of functioning (Miller-Perrin & Perrin, 1999).

Although poverty alone does not explain child neglect, it is certainly a risk factor (Garbarino & Collins, 1999). Children from low income families (i.e., those earning under $15,000 per year) were over 40 times more likely to be neglected than children from families earning over $30,000 per year (Sedlack & Broadhurst, 1996). While neglect may be more easily detected among poor families—because, in those cases, there is more likely inappropriate dress, evidence of malnutrition, and the like—it is important to note that emotional neglect occurs across all socioeconomic groups.

Child neglect is the most frequently reported type of child maltreatment, with over half of all substantiated child victims experiencing neglect (DHHS, 1999; Wang & Daro, 1998). Ironically, this type of maltreatment is often the least likely to be the focus of research or clinical attention. Most of the neglect statistics are taken from national incidence studies. Neglect occurs most often among children under the age of 8, with the largest percentage (34%) being children under the age of 3. Boys and girls appear to be at equal risk for child neglect (DHHS, 1999), however, boys seem to be at particular risk for emotional neglect (Sedlack & Broadhurst, 1996). Children from larger families (i.e., four or more children) also appear to be at greater risk for child neglect, being two to three times more likely to experience physical and/or educational neglect, as compared to children from smaller families (Sedlack & Broadhurst, 1996).

Contrary to the case of offenders in other forms of child maltreatment, females are more commonly charged with neglect than males (Sedlack &

Broadhurst, 1996). This finding is misleading, however, because it does not account for the numerous fathers who have ultimately neglected their children and families by abandoning them. Father abandonment produces a greater percentage of female-headed households, which are disproportionately represented in this maltreatment category.

Other characteristics of caregivers who neglect their children include having little to no social support, having poor social skills, and having a limited understanding of parenting norms (Black & Dubowitz, 1999). Research has also shown a higher rate of depression or depressive symptoms among mothers of neglected children, and these caregivers have a tendency to engage in role reversal with their children, allowing the child to parent him/herself and the parent (Black & Dubowitz, 1999).

Witnessing Domestic Violence

John was sitting in Mr. Cowan's first-grade class, trying hard to complete a reading worksheet. He struggled to keep his mind on his work, but even the slightest movements and sounds in the classroom and hallway startled him. At times, John's mind would wander back to last night, and he would experience a cold chill as he recalled the images of his father repeatedly punching his mother in the face while she struggled to get away or protect herself. John had seen it all as he sat statue-like in a strategic position at the top of the stairs. Mr. Cowan's stern direction to "get busy" brought his focus back to his worksheet, but he felt so tired. He knew it was because his parents' fighting had ended in the early morning hours and that it had been difficult for him to shut out the images and fall asleep. This was not the first time that John had witnessed violence in his home, and he knew it would probably not be the last. John only wished he could block out these thoughts and feelings and finish his worksheet so he could go to recess because recess was the only time he could forget about what was going on at home and just be a first grader.

The final type of maltreatment that will be reviewed and referenced in this book is children's witnessing marital conflict or domestic violence. Actual incidence rates and characteristics of children who experience this form of child maltreatment are unknown, as this category of maltreatment is not usually defined, or reported separately, in national incidence studies. Previously forgotten or categorized under "other forms of maltreatment" or psychological maltreatment, exposure to domestic violence is now being recognized as child maltreatment in its own right (Horton, Cruise, Graybill, & Cornett, 1999). Researchers have begun to examine the incidence, prevalence, and negative effects of witnessing domestic violence among children (Cummings & Davies, 1994; Jaffe, Sudermann, & Reitzel, 1992; Margolin, 1998). Based upon the number of women battered each year and the average number of children in those violent homes, it is estimated that between 3 and 10 million children are exposed to marital violence each year (Gelles & Straus, 1988; Margolin, 1998).

Domestic violence is a form of maltreatment to which children are exposed indirectly; they are the unintended victims. Although most intimate partners occasionally disagree or have "heated arguments," domestic violence is a pattern of behaviors between these individuals that involves physical, verbal, and/or sexual assaults, threats, or coercion. Domestic violence occurs most commonly with males aggressing against females (Jaffe et al., 1992; Margolin, 1998). Exposure to this type of violence is often chronic and severe, and occurs in the home, which is supposed to be a place of safety and trust for a child (Margolin, 1998). Even though many parents believe they protect their children from this type of violence by "arguing" after the children have gone to bed or when the children are believed to be out of sight, most children have at least heard, if not observed, the violence at these times. Some children experience the violence more directly by being forced to watch the encounters or having to report on the actions of the mother while the father was gone (Edleson, 1999b). Still others may only see the aftermath of the assault (e.g., black and swollen eyes, cuts or scrapes, broken bones, police intervention, the arrest of the father), or at the very least these children experience the tension in the home and are aware of the nonverbal hostility displayed by the adults.

Child witnesses to domestic violence are believed, by many, to be victims of some form of psychological neglect or psychological abuse. They might be considered by CPS as being "at risk for harm," as they may physically and/or psychologically be "in harm's way," living in a violent household. Increasingly, however, some (e.g., Edleson, 1999a) are questioning the wisdom of considering exposure to domestic violence as child abuse in a legal sense, and thereby having CPS involved in these situations. While not minimizing the potential negative effects on some child witnesses, Edleson (1999a) has pointed out some unintended consequences of this approach. For example, he notes that "battered women" frequently stay with their abusive partners to protect their children because they correctly understand that they (and their children) are in most danger immediately after leaving a batterer, and, if a divorce occurred, the children would likely have unsupervised visitation with this violent partner. Too often, however, women in these situations are misunderstood and charged with "failure to protect" their children (a charge rarely applied to their violent partner). In some cases children are even removed from the mother's custody, adding additional trauma and loss. Thus, Edleson (1999a) argues, in some cases children and their mothers are being revictimized by the very system designed to protect them. While the appropriate legal and child protection response might be controversial, exposure to domestic violence clearly can be traumatic and interfere with a child's development. Thus, clinically, exposure to domestic violence is a form of child maltreatment.

INCIDENCE AND PREVALENCE

There has been considerable debate over the definitions of maltreatment. For example, should the definitions include only actions that have resulted in observable harm, or should they be extended to include behaviors that endanger the lives of children but have yet to cause observable damage (English, 1998)? A child who is slapped several times in the face by a parent but has no physical bruises or marks would not be counted as physically abused under a narrow definition of harm but would certainly be considered endangered.

These different definitions and standards lead to variations in incidence and prevalence figures. Incidence refers to the number of cases of child maltreatment that occur during a specified time period (e.g., 1 year), whereas prevalence is a cumulative figure, referring to the number of individuals who have experienced at least one act of child maltreatment over some course of time (e.g., their childhood) (English, 1998; Wyncoop, Capps, & Priest, 1995). A recent national incidence study estimated that 3,195,000 children were reported as abused or neglected in 1997 (Wang & Daro, 1998). At approximately 1 million confirmed cases, this yielded a substantiated rate of 15 victims per every 1,000 children in the United States during that year, an 18% increase since 1990 (Wang & Daro, 1998). Reports made are either confirmed/substantiated or not substantiated/unfounded, but the distinction is not as simple as maltreatment actually occurring or not. Maltreatment reports may not be substantiated for numerous reasons, including a lack of information (e.g., the child is vague about who was abusive, and no one else can corroborate), reported situations in which the child is no longer at risk (e.g., an abusive boyfriend has moved out of state), or errors committed by CPS (Zellman & Faller, 1996). Therefore, many reported cases of maltreatment simply cannot be confirmed but may have still occurred and have still been harmful to the child.

Child neglect is the most common type of child maltreatment, with more than half (54%) of victims in 1997 experiencing some form of neglect (Wang & Daro, 1998). In the same report 22% of the victimized children suffered physical abuse, 8% sexual abuse, 4% emotional abuse, and 12% other forms of maltreatment (Wang & Daro, 1998), with many children experiencing more than one form of abuse. These incidence figures are clearly an underestimate of the actual number of cases of child maltreatment. Reasons for this include children not being able to report their abuse, the maltreatment never being discovered, or not having enough evidence of known cases of abuse not being reported, to substantiate a report. Prevalence figures confirm that the majority of child maltreatment cases are never reported to social service agencies or other professionals.

Prevalence estimates are most commonly drawn from self-report research and may vary based upon operational definitions of the various types of abuse, characteristics of the sample, and response rates. Although self-report and retrospective survey research has been criticized for potentially assessing "false memories" or exaggerating the number of cases of childhood maltreatment, some researchers (della Femina, Yeager, & Lewis, 1990; Williams, 1994) have posited that adults with abusive pasts are more likely to deny or minimize their experiences, resulting in an underestimation of maltreatment cases.

Retrospective surveys of adults find that between 16% and 19% report experiencing some degree of physical abuse during childhood (Schaaf & McCanne, 1998; Wind & Silvern, 1992). Similarly, prevalence estimates for sexual abuse are that at least 15–20% of females and 5–10% of males are victimized sometime during their childhood (Finkelhor, 1994; Gorey & Leslie, 1997). A 1995 Gallup poll found slightly higher rates, with 23% of adults surveyed reporting at least one instance of childhood sexual abuse. These rates, when projected to the population at that time, would have yielded a rate 10 times higher than that officially reported (English, 1998), again documenting that reported rates are just "the tip of the iceberg."

There are limited prevalence data on the other forms of abuse. Definitions of emotional abuse, neglect, and exposure to domestic violence are somewhat more ambiguous, and these forms have received significantly less research attention to date. There are, however, a few notable findings. For example, disturbing results from the National Family Violence Survey indicated that 63% of parents (from a survey of 6,000 households) reported using either verbal (e.g., insulting or swearing) or nonverbal (e.g., sulking) emotionally abusive forms of interaction with their children during the preceding year (Vissing, Straus, Gelles, & Harrop, 1991). Surveys of adults find that between 13% and 35% recall witnessing domestic violence between their parents or parental figures (Maker, Kemmelmeier, & Peterson, 1998; Straus, 1992).

While the separate incidence and prevalence figures for each type of maltreatment alone are alarming, many children endure multiple forms of abuse or neglect. For example, between 45% and 70% of the children who witness domestic violence also experience physical abuse (Rosenbaum & O'Leary, 1981; Salzinger, 1999). There is also an increased risk for sexual abuse, with these child witnesses being 12 to 14 times more likely to be molested by the mother's partner than nonwitnesses (McCloskey, Figueredo, & Koss, 1995).

RISK FACTORS

Although children of both genders and all ages, racial and ethnic groups, and socioeconomic status (SES) levels experience child maltreatment, there are some characteristics of parents/caregivers, children, and families that increase the risk of maltreatment (see Table 1.3 for a summary). General risk

TABLE 1.3. Risk Factors for Child Maltreatment

Parent/caregiver characteristics	Child characteristics	Family characteristics
Low self-esteem	Young age	Low SES
Feelings of inadequacy	Difficult temperament/	Single-parent
Depression	behaviors	households
Anxiety	Physical or mental	Large family size
Substance abuse/dependence	disabilities	Social isolation
Poor impulse control or anger control	Premature infants	Less cohesion among
Parental stress		members
Other psychological impairments		More verbal and
(e.g., personality disorders)		physical conflict
Young age		among members
Lower education		
External locus of control		
Perceive more negative child behaviors		
Attribute more blame and hostile intent to child behavior		
Less empathic toward children		
Intergenerational child maltreatment or domestic violence		
Impaired attachments with children		
Deficits in knowledge of child development		
Inappropriate expectations of children		
Deficits in parenting skills		

Note. Information for this table was obtained from the following sources: Dubowitz (1999); English (1998); Miller-Perrin and Perrin (1999); and Milner (1998).

factors for abuse and neglect will be discussed in this section, as risk factors for specific types of maltreatment (e.g., gender of child and perpetrator, age of child) were previously presented. Much is still unknown regarding how each risk factor alone contributes to the overall likelihood of abuse or neglect, and even less is known about how risk factors interact or are influenced by protective factors (English, 1999). For example, most people who have lower incomes do not mistreat their children, but poverty is often associated with more stress and social isolation in families, and it appears that this combination often leads to higher levels of child maltreatment (English, 1998, 1999; Milner, 1998).

Parent/Caregiver Characteristics

There is no universal psychological profile for an abusive parent, although parental risk factors have been identified. Empirical investigations have noted psychological impairments (e.g., low self-esteem, poor impulse control, antisocial personality disorder) or emotional problems (e.g., depression, anxiety) among many parent perpetrators; however, the majority of these offenders (less than 10%) are not severely disturbed or psychotic (for reviews, see Dubowitz, 1999; Miller-Perrin & Perrin, 1999; and Milner, 1998).

The emotional concerns experienced by most perpetrating parents, however, contribute to their abilities to attach to and effectively parent their children. Insecure attachments between parents and children have been noted as a risk factor for physical abuse, neglect, and psychological abuse (Kolko, 1992). This insecure attachment may be the result of inconsistent responding or the lack of responsiveness from the caregiver. An additional psychological disturbance most commonly noted by CPS caseworkers when investigating reports of child maltreatment is parental substance abuse (Wang & Daro, 1998). Substance abuse may also impair parents' abilities to meet the physical and emotional needs of their children and to form secure attachments.

A parent's own childhood experience of maltreatment has also been noted as a risk factor for physical abuse and neglect (English, 1998; Salzinger, 1999). There has been substantial literature on the intergenerational transmission of physical abuse among parents who were physically abused (for reviews, see Miller-Perrin & Perrin, 1999; Milner, 1998; and Youngblade & Belsky, 1990) and more recently among parents who were sexually abused (DiLillo, Tremblay, & Peterson, 2000). Some parents may emulate the physically harsh parenting style they experienced. They have come to view violence as an acceptable method of expressing anger or disapproval (Jaffe, Wolfe, & Wilson, 1990). Certainly many parents who were maltreated during childhood will not repeat such patterns with their own children. The cycle of abuse and neglect is more likely to continue when abused parents are faced with other risk factors.

Psychological impairments, attachment patterns, and personal histories of abuse may contribute directly to the cognitive risk factors associated with abusive and neglectful parents. Thirty-nine percent of federally appointed CPS specialists noted parental capacity and lack of effective parenting skills as common problems among reported families (Wang & Daro, 1998). For example, a parent who does not feel good about him/herself and has not had good parenting role models may lack an understanding of child development and parenting skills. This, in turn, may result in parents having inappropriate expectations of their child and experiencing greater upset when these expectations are not met. Maltreating parents are more likely to use punishment, threats, or coercion in an attempt to control their children, and are less likely to use reasoning or positive reinforcers (Milner, 1998; Salzinger, 1999). Abusive parents have also been found to have more negative attitudes toward parenting than nonabusive parents do and to perceive more negative behavior in their children (English, 1998; Milner, 1998; Salzinger, 1999). Again, this may result in greater parental distress, and, when accompanied by a lack of effective parenting skills or poor impulse control, child maltreatment may occur.

Younger parents are more at risk for abusing their children (DHHS, 1999; Miller-Perrin & Perrin, 1999). Lack of parenting skills and emotional immaturity often place these parents at greater risk for harming their children. Further, females may be slightly more at risk for abusing their children, but this is likely an artifact of father absence and children being more commonly in the care of their mother. Thus, these issues are important considerations in the school-based prevention of child maltreatment (which is discussed in Chapter 7).

Child Characteristics

Although children are not to blame for their own victimization, there are characteristics of the individual child that may place him or her at greater risk of harm. Children who suffer from low self-esteem or are passive or emotionally needy (e.g., overly eager to please or fit in, clingy) may be more vulnerable to sexual abuse (Finkelhor, 1994). Further, children with difficult or irritable temperaments, which may include more whining, demanding, or aggressive behaviors and trouble adapting to change, are more likely to be abused or neglected (English, 1998; Miller-Perrin & Perrin, 1999). Researchers have also suggested that premature infants and children with disabilities (e.g., learning disability, speech or language delay or impairment, emotional/behavioral disturbance, physical impairments) are at greater risk for maltreatment (Dubowitz, 1999; English, 1998; Miller-Perrin & Perrin, 1999; Morgan, 1994). Children with these characteristics may create more stress for already vulnerable parents, and this may ultimately contribute to greater emotional distance between the parent and child. Thus, the child's characteristics and the parent's response style, which may include hyperarousal and impulsiveness, create a reciprocal relationship that may set the stage for later maltreatment. Yet, not all premature infants or difficult babies are mistreated, so it appears to be the cumulative stress on the parent and his or her response style that determines whether a child with these characteristics will be harmed.

Younger children are also more at risk. In a recent incidence study, children under the age of 7 were more likely to be abused or neglected (DHHS, 1999). Children under the age of 4 were also more likely to be fatally injured or killed. Again, it is obviously not simply the age of the child that leads to mistreatment, but rather aspects of young children (such as their crying and dependence) may combine with other risk factors of the caregiver or family to produce increased risk.

Family Characteristics

Lower family socioeconomic status is a commonly reported risk factor for all types of child maltreatment. Although child maltreatment occurs among all socioeconomic levels, children from lower-SES families are more often the victims. In 1996 Sedlack and Broadhurst reported that children from families with annual incomes below $15,000 were 22 times more likely to experience some form of maltreatment than children from families that earned $30,000 or more per year. Family income was the strongest correlate of incidence across all categories of maltreatment (Sedlack & Broadhurst, 1996). Victims from lower income families had the greatest likelihood of experiencing all types of neglect and serious injury or death (Sedlack & Broadhurst, 1996). Although resources are necessary to meet a family's basic needs and may create more stress and a greater likelihood of neglect when lacking, families who have lower incomes often have other related problems that may contribute to child maltreatment (e.g., lack of social support, substance abuse, unemployment, limited education).

Single-parent households are often associated with lower SES and have been found to be a risk factor for child maltreatment. In the NIS-3 study children from single-parent homes were found to be at a 77% greater risk of physical abuse and at a higher risk for all types of neglect (87% physical, 74% emotional, 220% educational) than those from two-parent homes (Sedlack & Broadhurst, 1996). Additionally, children from single-parent homes were at a greater risk of suffering serious or moderate injuries (Sedlack & Broadhurst, 1996). Single parents may not have the financial and emotional supports needed to act as a buffer to the emotional strains and stresses of parenting, thus making them a more at-risk group.

Low-income and single-parent families are also more likely to experience social isolation and to lack a social support network. This, in turn, may contribute to higher levels of parental stress, lack of knowledge regarding parenting skills and community resources, lack of help in caring for their children, and poorer parental psychological functioning. Such parents have few, if any, buffers for the stress and burdens they are experiencing, and it is the children who are made to pay the price. Family isolation may also prevent children from finding good role models and becoming involved in constructive activities, and in worst-case scenarios it may help maintain the family's secret regarding child maltreatment. Parents who are at risk for abusing or neglecting their children may also be mistrusting of others and decline assistance when offered for fear of being discovered. Yet, it is this social support that has been found to mediate the relationships between poverty and high parental stress and poor parenting (Salzinger, 1999).

Family size has also been suggested as a risk factor in child maltreatment. The larger the family, the fewer the resources there may be to spread to each member. These resources include not only material possessions such as food and clothing but also emotional resources such as time and attention. As family size increases, the risk for children to become abused or neglected also increases (DHHS, 1999; Milner, 1998).

Although these risk factors do not often occur in isolation and may not alone be a precursor to abuse, one should be aware of them and how they contribute to child maltreatment. One certainty is that abusive families are often "struggling with a combination of stresses that they experience as overwhelming and for which they do not have the coping skills" (Morgan, 1994, p. 133).

CONSEQUENCES OF CHILD MALTREATMENT

There is no single "child abuse syndrome," no one specific response pattern for children who endure single or multiple forms of maltreatment. There is, however, evidence of a variety of psychological correlates among child and adolescent victims. Some victims will not exhibit any initial or long-term damaging effects (Browne & Finkelhor, 1986; Holmes & Slap, 1998; Jaffe et al., 1990; Margolin, 1998; Rind, Tromovitch, & Bauserman, 1998), while others may have delayed effects that do not emerge until adolescence or adulthood, a phenomenon referred to as the "sleeper effect." There is great variety in the extent and types of symptoms exhibited by maltreated children.

Physiological Effects

Direct physical injuries are perhaps the most obvious effects of child maltreatment and are most often associated with physical abuse. For example, physical abuse may produce injuries to a child's skin (such as bruises, welts, abrasions, puncture wounds, burns, and scaldings), skeletal structure (such as skull and bone fractures and dislocations), or internal organs (such as brain damage, internal bleeding, or ruptured organs) (Gelardo & Sanford, 1987; Miller-Perrin & Perrin, 1999).

Sexual abuse, in a small minority of cases, may also produce physical injuries, including bladder injuries, rectal and vaginal tears or bruising, and lacerations on genitalia (Bates, 1980; Brassard, Tyler, & Kehle, 1983; Morgan, 1994). Genital pain or itching, sexually transmitted diseases, and pregnancy are other noted physical effects. Yet, clear physical indicators of sexual abuse are the exception rather than the norm. Child victims may, however, experience other somatic complaints (e.g., headaches, stomachaches, irritable bowel syndrome) or may regress from once mastered developmental milestones, such as becoming enuretic or encopretic after mastering toileting (Kendall-Tackett, Williams, & Finkelhor, 1993; Kendall-Tackett, 2000; Morgan, 1994). Victims of child sexual abuse may also experience disturbances in their eating and sleeping patterns (e.g., insomnia, night terrors) (Beitchman, Zucker, Hood, DaCosta, & Akman, 1991; Kendall-Tackett, 2000; Vevier & Tharinger, 1986).

Children who are victims of neglect certainly experience physical symptoms. Poor weight gain, delayed growth, and varying degrees of malnutrition are some examples (Cantwell, 1980; Helfer, 1987). Since a vast proportion of the brain develops prior to the age of 6, physical and emotional neglect may have critical negative effects on neural development (Morgan, 1994). Unfortunately, this growth may not be regained outside of this critical period. Neglected children are also prone to frequent illness. While the illnesses may not be serious, they are often chronic (Helfer, 1987). Nonorganic failure to thrive (NOFTT) syndrome (i.e., failure over time to grow to accepted standards for height, weight, and development but not due to organic deficits) has been used to describe children who have been physically or emotionally neglected (Gaudin, 1999; Helfer, 1987). The success of interventions to prevent the long-term deficits of NOFTT depends on caregiver cooperation and involvement; otherwise, these children may have developmental deficits that affect them across several dimensions (e.g., cognitive, physical, emotional) (Gaudin, 1999).

Similar to children who experience sexual abuse or neglect, children who witness domestic violence display a variety of psychosomatic problems, including headaches and stomachaches (Carlson, 1984). High levels of stress-related disorders, including asthma, diarrhea, ulcers, and other intestinal problems, have been documented among these victims (Carlson, 1984; Margolin, 1998). Regressions in toileting and language, along with eating problems and sleeping difficulties, such as insomnia, sleepwalking, and nightmares, have also been observed (Carlson, 1984; Margolin, 1998). In addition to the indirect effects this form of maltreatment may have on children's physical health, there is the direct risk of intentional or accidental physical injury should a child become involved in the adult conflict (Carlson, 1984).

Another physiological response to victimization that has been found across the different types of maltreatment is chronic hyperarousal (van der Kolk, 1989; Kendall-Tackett, 2000; Terr, 1991). Through the process of sensitization victims have generalized the stress response they experienced during their victimization to more general life stressors (van der Kolk, 1989; Kendall-Tackett, 2000). Thus, victims of maltreatment often respond abnormally to new everyday stressors by engaging in a fight-or-flight response that demands action rather than thought (van der Kolk, 1989). Functioning in this chronic state of hyperarousal is believed to be related to somatic symptoms and, more recently, alterations in the brain (van der Kolk, 1989; Kendall-Tackett, 2000).

Recent research has begun to explore other biological effects of child maltreatment, such as changes in brain structures, hormone types and levels, growth patterns, and pain threshold levels (for a review, see Kaplan, Pelcovitz, & Labruna, 1999). Others are investigating child maltreatment as a risk factor for physiological problems (e.g., irritable bowel syndrome, fibromyalgia) (Kendall-Tackett, 2000; Walker et al., 1997).

Affective Effects

Victims of maltreatment frequently have effects beyond physical injuries or neurological damage; there is often great emotional distress that contributes to ongoing difficulties in psychological functioning and interpersonal relationships. Children who have been maltreated often display externalizing and/or internalizing symptomology. It is the externalizing symptoms (i.e., acting-out behaviors) that typically receive the most attention from school personnel, and these will be addressed further in the next section; however, children displaying internalizing symptomology need to receive equal attention to ensure some type of intervention for these children as well.

Internalizing symptoms commonly found among children who have been abused, neglected, or witnessed domestic violence include withdrawal, depression, anxiety, fear, hypervigilance, anger, low self-esteem, and blunted or restricted affect (Browne & Finkelhor, 1986; Erickson & Egeland, 1987; Gaudin, 1999; Gross & Keller, 1992; Haskett & Kistner, 1991; Kaufman & Cicchetti, 1989; Kolko, 1992; Youngblade & Belsky, 1990).

Abused children may learn that by being unheard and unseen they are at less risk of harm. As a result, they may begin to withdraw, deny their own feelings and opinions, and demonstrate more blunted affect (Peterson & Urquiza, 1993). Neglected children may also develop a restricted affective range because they have not had interpersonal relationships that model emotional expression or mirror their personal effect on others.

Children who have been maltreated often feel different from others and struggle with understanding that they are not responsible for their victimization. Many may interpret the maltreatment as their fault and believe that they deserve it, which ultimately lowers self-esteem. Other children who lack support and attention from caregivers feel invisible and do not develop a strong sense of who they are or feel negatively about themselves. Children who have lowered self-esteem may then approach social experiences with negative expectations, and, if these expectations are met, the child feels even worse about him- or herself (Kaufman & Cicchetti, 1989).

Children's attributional styles may be related to their internalizing symptomatology. For example, stable internal attributional styles have been found among sexual abuse victims. Thus, they may experience a great sense of shame or blame because they believe they had some responsibility for or control over what happened. This may be accompanied by a sense of powerlessness in their environment and a perception of themselves as "damaged goods" (Bergner, 1990). This attributional style has been linked to depression among survivors. On the other hand, children subjected to emotional abuse may feel that unstable external influences control the outcomes in their lives. Thus, they feel that they have little impact or control in changing what happers and are left feeling sad and helpless.

Children from violent or abusive homes may display extreme fear as a result of living in such a violent, unpredictable environment. They may also display more hypervigilance (i.e., greater sensitivity to noise, movement, adult mood changes). Some children use this heightened sensitivity to avoid or emotionally prepare themselves for the next abusive episode, while others have developed such a keen awareness of their environment that they are able to escape relatively unnoticed or even sneak resources (e.g., food, clothing).

Many of these internalizing symptoms have also been noted as long-term consequences. Researchers and clinicians who work with adolescent and adult survivors of child maltreatment indicate that these survivors often exhibit depression, anxiety, feelings of isolation and stigma, hyperarousal, and low self-esteem (Browne & Finkelhor, 1986; Gaudin, 1999; Holmes & Slap, 1998; Margolin, 1998; Wind & Silvern, 1992).

One additional affective response to maltreatment worthy of note is anger. Anger, understandably, is another emotion commonly experienced by children who have been maltreated. Some children may be angry with their perpetrators, while others are also angry with the individuals who failed to prevent the abuse or neglect or who failed to believe the victim upon disclosure or discovery. This generalized anger toward others may lead to behavioral and interpersonal difficulties.

Behavioral/Interpersonal Effects

Instead of, or in addition to, internalizing symptoms, children who have been maltreated may display externalizing behavior patterns. Behaviors may range from being clingy and overly dependent to outward defiance. The most common externalizing behavior, even among preschoolers, is instrumental aggression (Erikson & Egeland, 1987; Kaplan et al., 1999; Kendall-Tackett et al., 1993; Vissing et al., 1991). Clearly, not all children who have been maltreated become aggressive. Just as in other pathologies, there may be a temperamental or genetic predisposition toward aggression or resiliency. However, a child's impaired attachment with an abusive caregiver may leave the child expecting hurt or rejection to be part of his/her interactions with others. Maltreated children are missing a meaningful, consistent relationship through which they can meet their personal needs. Additionally, living with aggressive adult models and experiencing physical assaults at the hands of one's parents may also result in more anger and impulsivity and alter the child's perceptions of pain in him/herself and others (Lewis, 1992). In response to the powerlessness children may feel regarding their maltreatment or in response to their unheard cries for help, some children may identify with the aggressor and bully or aggress against peers or adults (Finkelhor, 1988).

The aggressive approach these children take with peers may be extended to relationships with adults as well. This may take the form of passive noncompliance or outward defiance. Adolescents may become more physically aggressive toward parents and other adults, and some have been found to be abusive in their dating relationships (Maker et al., 1998; Wolfe, Wekerle, Reitzel-Jaffe, & Lefebvre, 1998).

Aggressive tendencies may develop into more serious conduct problems in adolescence, including fighting, property offenses, and other criminality (Beitchman et al., 1991; Edleson, 1999b; Kolko, 1992; Margolin, 1998; Salzinger, 1999). Adolescents may also turn their aggression inward, which is reflected in the links between child maltreatment and suicidal and other self-injurious behavior, alcohol and drug abuse, and cigarette smoking (Beitchman et al., 1991; Kaplan et al., 1999; Kolko, 1992; Osofsky & Scheeringa, 1997). One striking finding by Mullen and colleagues was that emotional abuse victims were 12 times more likely to attempt suicide than their nonabused peers (Mullen, Martin, Anderson, Romans, & Herbison, 1996).

Given these symptom patterns, it is not surprising that children who have been maltreated have disrupted peer relations (Gaudin, 1999; Kaplan et al., 1999; Peterson & Urquiza, 1993). In fact, the social-peer domain, which involves reciprocal relationships of sharing and nonexploitation, is perhaps the most affected area for abused and neglected children (Jaffe et al., 1992; Goodman & Rosenberg, 1987; Kolko, 1992; Peterson & Urquiza, 1993). Their lack of understanding that there must be give and take in any relationship results in their displaying poor impulse control or having difficulty delaying gratification (Peterson & Urquiza, 1993). Maltreated children typically have a number of social skill deficits, including difficulty in making friends and limited prosocial behaviors (e.g., sharing, initiating, smiling). They also lack effective social problem solving or conflict resolution skills, which means they are more likely to use aggression as a coping method (Goodman & Rosenberg, 1987; Miller-Perrin & Perrin, 1999; Wolfe et al., 1998).

Some maltreated children may misinterpret the intent of peer behavior to be more hostile and will respond with either aggression or resistance (Kaplan et al., 1999; Youngblade & Belsky, 1990). Yet, for others the internalizing symptoms of fear, mistrust, and negative self-perceptions interfere with the development and maintenance of friendships. As a result, these children may exhibit greater dependency on adults and demonstrate a need for an unusual degree of reassurance (Brassard et al., 1983).

Further, maltreated children are believed to have impaired empathic abilities. For example, physically abused children often respond to peer distress with aggression (Kolko, 1992; Youngblade & Belsky, 1990). This difficulty empathizing with others makes it difficult for these maltreated children to take another child's perspective or understand the impact of their own behavior on others (Goodman & Rosenberg, 1987). Therefore, even at very young ages, peers find children who have been abused or neglected to be less desirable playmates, and thus these children continue to be at risk for peer rejection (Haskett & Kistner, 1991).

Abuse-Specific Behavior

Most of the previously mentioned consequences are not specific to any subtype of maltreatment. However, developmentally inappropriate sexualized behavior is a symptom specific to, and most predictive of, sexual abuse (Beitchman et al., 1991; Kendall-Tackett et al., 1993; James & Burch, 1999). Sexually abused children may develop an increased, excessive interest in, and a preoccupation or "obsession" with, sexuality, which may be manifested in a number of ways, including precocious sexual play, excessive masturbation, sexually aggressive behavior toward peers or adults, and age-inappropriate sexual knowledge and language (Berliner & Rawlings, 1991; Johnson & Friend, 1995). Adolescent sexual difficulties include sexual dissatisfaction, indiscriminate sexual behavior, and an increased risk for revictimization (Beitchman et al., 1991; Kendall-Tackett et al., 1993). (Information to guide educators in the identification of sexual behavior problems at school will be presented in the next chapter.)

Some clinicians and researchers believe that sexualized behavior among abused children may be an attempt to gain control or mastery over what has happened to them through reenacting their own abuse (van der Kolk, 1989; Terr, 1991). Other children may come to believe that sex is equated with love or that sex and aggression are paired, so they, in turn, express these needs to others accordingly (Finkelhor, 1988).

Academic Effects

In addition to the behavioral and emotional consequences of child maltreatment, academic problems are also frequent. Sudden changes in academic performance are common among victims of child maltreatment, as are more chronic school problems, including poor school achievement, failing grades, increased risk for retention or referrals for special education services, truancy, and dropping out (Eckenrode, Laird, & Doris, 1993; Erickson & Egeland, 1987; Leiter & Johnsen, 1997; Tower, 1992). Although children who have suffered from all forms of maltreatment may be at risk to experience problems in the academic arena, children who have been neglected were found to have the lowest academic skills, and these deficits remained even after controlling for SES (Eckenrode et al., 1993; Kurtz, Gaudin, Wodarski, & Howing, 1993). Academic problems may be noticed as early as preschool or kindergarten, occur primarily in the areas of reading, language, and math, and may place maltreated children at risk for retention at a rate twice that of their nonmaltreated classmates (Cantwell, 1980; Eckenrode et al., 1993; Kaplan et al., 1999; Kurtz et al., 1993).

There are multiple explanations for such academic difficulties. Clearly, emotional factors are critical considerations. As with John in the opening vignettes, it is often difficult for a child who is withdrawn, depressed, and having difficulty concentrating—due to the distress of recent abuse or the fear of potential future abuse—to learn. Further, the academic careers of maltreated children are often marked by considerable discontinuity, owing to frequent moves, school transfers, and absenteeism (Kolko, 1992).

Alternative or additional explanations may also apply. For example, if physical abuse involves head injuries, intellectual impairment may be a direct consequence (Gelardo & Sanford, 1987). Children who are hungry or malnourished, have medical conditions not addressed by the family, or need special resources (e.g., glasses or hearing aids) that are not provided or replaced when lost or broken (Tower, 1992) may have to struggle harder in an attempt to keep up with schoolwork.

Indirectly, abuse or neglect may diminish a child's curiosity about the world and stifle his or her motivation for independence and autonomy, which ultimately impedes the learning process (Salzinger, 1999). The child may lack a psychologically available parent who will provide the encouragement, participation, and responsiveness to school activities and achievements required for success (Helfer, 1987).

Additionally, the behavior problems many maltreated children display will often interrupt the instruction a child receives. Disciplinary problems (e.g., suspensions or expulsions) resulting from these behaviors may also increase academic difficulties.

Summary of Consequences

Consequences of child maltreatment vary in type and severity across children. A range of physiological, emotional, social/behavioral, and academic difficulties are common. These symptoms may represent children's "attempt to negotiate the trauma themselves" (Gil, 1991; Terr, 1991; van der Kolk, 1989).

FACTORS MEDIATING THE CONSEQUENCES OF CHILD MALTREATMENT

While a range of negative outcomes are possible, they are not inevitable or invariable for mistreated children. If maltreated children do experience symptoms, the symptoms may vary in type and severity. Factors thought to mediate the impact of child maltreatment include child characteristics, pre-abuse family functioning, aspects of the abuse experience, cognitive interpretation and coping strategies used, and response and support from others (see Table 1.4).

Empirical evidence for some of these factors is inconsistent, which suggests that other factors may actually mediate the trauma or more likely that some combination or interaction of these factors determines the outcome for each victim. At times, these factors have been found to function in a counter-intuitive manner. Force, for example, is generally thought to be more predictive of trauma; however, in some cases, abuse involving force and even the use of a weapon, while certainly distressing, may help clarify for a victim of sexual abuse who is the offender and who is the victim. Situations involving "nurturing perpetrators" who do not need to use violence may be less dramatic and traumatic in the moment, but may create long-term doubt, confusion, and guilt for the survivor who is left wondering, "Why didn't I stop him? Was he right? Did I like it, want it, ask for it? Am I dirty?"

Two examples may help to further illustrate the inconsistent influence of force on recovery. First, Hindman (1999) describes the story of two young

---

TABLE 1.4. Mediating Factors of Child Maltreatment

Child characteristics

♦ Age at onset of the abuse or neglect
♦ Gender
♦ Level of cognitive functioning

Preabuse family functioning

♦ Quality of the parent–child relationship
♦ Emotional climate of the family
♦ The child's emotional/mental health functioning

Aspects of the abuse experience

♦ Severity
♦ Chronicity
♦ Exposure to multiple forms of maltreatment
♦ Biological and/or emotional relationship with the offender
♦ Level of threat or force involved

Coping strategies/cognitive interpretation

♦ Type of coping strategies used (i.e., problem-focused vs. emotion-focused)
♦ Powerlessness/learned helplessness
♦ Attribution of responsibility (i.e., self-blame vs. blaming offender)

Note. Information for this table was obtained from the following sources: Beitchman, Zucker, Hood, DaCosta, and Akman (1991); Browne and Finkelhor (1986); Edleson (1999b); Gaudin (1999); Gil (1991); and Miller-Perrin and Perrin (1999).

girls who were dropped off at the movies by their mother. A stranger approached them during the movie and sexually assaulted them at knifepoint. The theater staff and audience captured the man and provided the girls with emotional support, cheering when the man was arrested and giving the girls popcorn until their mother arrived. The mother immediately believed the children and was supportive of them. Although this scenario involved invasive sexual acts and force, factors thought to be predictive of the greatest trauma, the girls, while certainly upset, did not necessarily suffer severe or long-term symptoms. A second story is about a young girl who was given undivided positive attention by her older cousin, who also frequently "persuaded" her to perform sexual acts on him while on the way to the Dairy Queen. Due to the lack of clear force and the perceived "caring" she received, this girl had greater difficulty assigning responsibility for the abuse to the cousin and therefore kept the abuse a secret.

The use of force combined with postabuse factors (e.g., immediate disclosure and support of others) in the first example facilitated clear cognitions regarding who was the victim and who was the perpetrator and mediated healthy recoveries. However, the lack of clear force in the second example and the girl's perception that she "consented" to the sexual acts created more confusion for the victim and left her feeling as though she allowed the abuse to happen. She never disclosed the abuse to others, who could have provided her with the support and information necessary to alter her interpretation of the events.

These case examples further illustrate the importance of others' responses to abuse detection and disclosure and the provision of ongoing support. Support given by someone outside the family, including school personnel, may counter some of the negativity the child would otherwise experience (Hindman, 1999; Margolin, 1998). The presence of even one supportive person in a child's social network was found to help ameliorate the long-term consequences of maltreatment (Briere & Elliott, 1994; Margolin, 1998).

CONCLUSION

Child maltreatment clearly is a major social concern. Literally millions of children are victimized by physical abuse, sexual abuse, emotional abuse, neglect, and exposure to domestic violence, with many experiencing multiple forms. While families experiencing poverty, isolation, and other stress may be more at risk, child maltreatment occurs in all kinds of families; stereotypes are often inaccurate. While victims often keep their abuse or neglect a secret, the negative effects on their physical, emotional, behavioral, and academic functioning are often evident. However, there is no universal syndrome that would help school personnel detect a maltreated child. Symptoms vary and the impact of abuse or neglect may be mediated by the specific aspects of the experience, individual child and parent characteristics, the parent–child relationship, and the response and support of others. While this extensive information may be overwhelming and disturbing, its recitation here sets the stage for an *informed* school-based response.

◆◆◆

Identifying Abuse and Neglect

◆

Detecting abuse and neglect is a vital role that schools may usefully play in responding to child maltreatment. "The school is usually the only setting outside the home in which the child victim of intrafamilial sexual abuse regularly participates. Thus, the child's presence in school often constitutes the only opportunity for this form of sexual abuse to be detected, identified, and reported" (Vevier & Tharinger, 1986, pp. 293–294). While these remarks were made about sexual abuse specifically, they apply to much of child maltreatment. Schools truly do have a unique opportunity and responsibility.

Before considering specific indicators to be aware of, or step-by-step directions in how to respond to a child's disclosure, school personnel must consider some basic attitudes and assumptions about detecting abuse.

1. *A realistic view of prevalence rates is important.* First, to be prepared to detect abuse, one must be aware of the frequency of its occurrence. The incidence and prevalence rates discussed in the preceding chapter are sobering. Consider, again, just a few of them. One in four girls is sexually abused before she reaches 18 years of age (Finkelhor, 1994). At least 16% of children experience physical abuse. Neglect is even more common. Many other children—an estimated 3.3 million per year—are exposed to family violence (Gelles & Straus, 1988). These are but a few of the disturbing incidence and prevalence figures. Clearly, far too many children are secretly suffering abuse. School personnel, who see these children daily, have a commonsensical responsibility to assist in detecting and intervening to protect victims of maltreatment. To act otherwise would allow suffering to continue, with potentially serious negative consequences for these children, their families, and society at large. School personnel, to be prepared, must be realistic and fully cognizant that *child abuse really does happen in the lives of many students.*

School professionals must acknowledge their own feelings regarding these incidence rates (Vevier & Tharinger, 1986). Certainly, it can be overwhelming to consider that in each classroom there may be children who live in abusive homes. Denial is an understandable, albeit not helpful, response. As a school professional, one should realistically expect to encounter a number of abused children every year.

Certainly school personnel should avoid ever getting to the point that they "jump to abuse conclusions." A situation in which every bruise is thought to be the result of physical abuse, every sexual question an indicator of sexual abuse, and every sign of anxiety "evidence" of maltreatment would neither be helpful to anyone nor conducive to learning. School personnel must come to understand that child abuse and neglect are far too common to be dismissed out of hand. But jumping to conclusions too soon or going on "witch hunts," is also irresponsible.

2. *Being aware of the most common symptoms of abuse is helpful.* Commonly observed symptoms of maltreatment, while not conclusive singly or in isolation, are *indicators* of *possible* abuse (Gil, 1991). Such symptoms typically may indicate some level of distress or concern but are not necessarily specific to abuse. Thus, school professionals should not prematurely assume that any child who displays these symptoms has been abused. Lists of "indicators" or "effects," however, should prompt school professionals to consider possible abuse explanations for a child's behavior, affect, or school performance.

Accurate awareness of prevalence rates and potential symptoms of abuse should lead school personnel to consider abuse as a *possible* cause of some behaviors. For example, when a child is referred for an assessment because of his or her poor academic performance, does that school psychologist *consider* whether the child has adequate rest and nutrition before coming to school? When an adolescent female is refusing to dress for physical education does the coach *contemplate the possibility* that the student may be experiencing shame and discomfort regarding her body due to sexual abuse? When a kindergarten boy is extremely aggressive, does the teacher *wonder about* where he learned that behavior or what is behind the anger before developing a behavior modification plan? When a child is referred to school professionals for suspected attention-deficit/hyperactivity disorder (ADHD) due to an inability to concentrate, does anyone at school *ask the question* "Is there something that child is concentrating on . . . or working hard to forget?"

3. *School personnel are not child abuse detectives or investigators.* While school personnel may be in key positions to detect actual abuse or to respond to the disclosures of children, they are not detectives or investigative agents. State CPS (child protective services) departments exist to investigate potential instances of child maltreatment.

Children should be interviewed at school only in sufficient depth to determine whether a report, with key information regarding the alleged incident, should be forwarded to the child protection agency. School personnel are not in a position to determine whether or not an alleged incident actually occurred. Their role is to only determine if there is a reason to suspect a child may have been maltreated and, if so, to pass the matter along to the appropriate investigative authorities.

4. *Collaboration is key.* Recognizing possible abuse is not a role limited to school psychologists or social workers. In fact, one of the most important roles of those professionals may be in supporting teachers to use their own opportunities to identify students who may be being abused or neglected.

Teachers may be the first to recognize aggressive or withdrawn behavior or sudden changes in a student's demeanor. A school nurse might be the first to be aware of a pattern of unexplained bruises or other injuries. A school psychologist may uncover some suspicious response patterns in doing a psychoeducational evaluation. School administrators or social workers may have had more firsthand contact with parents. Free and open communication among school professionals may be important if child abuse is to be accurately detected. In many instances, one professional may have sufficient information to make a report independently. At other times, when school professionals share their separate lower-level concerns with one another, collectively they may believe they have reason to suspect. Such discussions should respect the confidentiality of all parties, and should clearly be on a "need-to-know basis."

Additionally, collaboration beyond the school is also important. The school personnel's relationships with families, particularly with nonoffending parents, remain critical (Tharinger & Horton, 1992). School practitioners should strive to develop positive relationships with the social service agencies in their community and specifically with child protection agencies. Schools and such agencies can work together in partnership, understanding and appreciating the unique role that each can play.

CONSIDERING POSSIBLE INDICATORS

With these assumptions in mind, school personnel are better prepared to consider possible indicators. Table 2.1 provides a list of common consequences of child maltreatment discussed in the previous chapter. Sensitive educators can pick up important *possible* signs of abuse by observing children at school, remembering that often the "recognition of child maltreatment is not based upon the detection of one or two clues, but rather on the recognition of a cluster of indicators that make up a composite" (Tower, 1992, p. 15).

Academic Factors

School personnel, especially teachers, have a particularly unique opportunity to observe a child's academic performance. Recall from Chapter 1 that chil-

TABLE 2.1. Consequences of Maltreatment Observed by School Personnel

Physical

- Repeated marks, cuts, bruises, or other injuries
- Frequent reports of "accidents" to explain obvious or serious injuries
- Frequent illnesses
- Somatic complaints—stomachaches, headaches, general aches and pains
- Regressive behaviors—tantruming, baby talk, thumb sucking, enuresis, encopresis
- Disturbances in eating behaviors—lack of appetite, gorging, significant weight loss or gain, hoarding or stealing food
- Consistently tired in class or low energy level
- Hyperarousal or hypervigilance—sensitivity to noise, movement, or adult mood changes
- Impaired vision or hearing, for which aids are not provided or replaced when broken
- Consistently poor hygiene and/or inappropriate dress

Behavioral

- Impulsiveness
- Verbal or physical aggressiveness
- Overly compliant or clingy
- Defiant acting out
- Fire setting
- Cruelty to animals
- Sexually problematic behaviors (e.g., excessive masturbation, promiscuity, age-inappropriate sexual language or knowledge)
- Substance abuse
- Delinquency/criminality
- Self-mutilation—cutting or burning oneself
- Suicide gestures
- Running away

Social and emotional

- Lack of interest in pleasurable activities
- Chronic depressed mood
- Socially isolated or withdrawn
- Low self-esteem
- Flat or blunted affect
- Dissociation—psychologically removing oneself from one's body, as evident in glazed eyes, blank stares, or delayed or absent responses
- General fear response to people, objects, or situations
- Nervousness or anxiety—as evident in fidgeting, difficulty in attending, or compulsive actions
- Impaired trust
- Social skill deficits—lack of prosocial behaviors, decreased empathy, inability to make friends
- Role reversal—child is acting in a parent role toward self and others

Learning difficulties

- Sudden change in academic performance
- Failing grades   *(continued)*

TABLE 2.1. *(continued)*

Learning difficulties *(cont.)*

♦ Low standardized test scores—especially in reading, language, and math
♦ Higher risk for retention or special education placement
♦ Frequent moves or transfers
♦ Impaired curiosity and creativity
♦ Difficulty in focusing or sustaining attention
♦ Truancy or absenteeism—may be to avoid feeling stigmatized or in order to feel safe

Note. Information for this table was obtained from the following sources: Beitchman, Zucker, Hood, DaCosta, and Akman (1991); Browne and Finkelhor (1986); Eckenrode, Laird, and Doris (1993); Erickson and Egeland (1987); Gil (1991); Jaffe, Sudermann, and Reitzel (1992); Kaplan, Pelcovitz, and Labruna (1999); Kendall-Tackett, Williams, and Finkelhor (1993); Kolko (1992); Kurtz, Gaudin, Wodarski, and Howing (1993); Leiter and Johnsen (1997); Margolin (1998); Miller-Perrin and Perrin (1999); Morgan (1994); Peterson and Urquiza (1993); Tower (1992); and Youngblade and Belsky (1990).

dren who have been abused or neglected, as a group, have lower grades, more suspensions, disciplinary referrals, and more grade repetitions. When children are having serious academic problems that cannot be explained by cognitive deficits or learning disabilities, abuse and/or neglect should be considered as (only) one possible explanation. In some cases even the cognitive deficits or learning disabilities may have resulted from abuse.

Difficulty in Concentrating

A common connection between child abuse and academic difficulties may well be head or brain injuries. At times, head injuries may result in an impaired ability to concentrate. At other times, the reason for concentration difficulties may be less neurological or physiological than emotional. It may simply be difficult for children who are being abused to concentrate; they have so many other, more pressing, things on their mind than the academic work before them. As one survivor of abuse explained, "It's like I have all this noise in my head and I can't think of other things. . . . All I thought about was what would happen or what had happened" (quoted in Nugent, Labram, & McLoughlin, 1998, p. 73).

Imagine the surreal experience students currently living in abusive homes must have, trying to focus on academic work. Consider the following hypothetical, yet realistic, example. Johnny hears the teacher scolding him. "Johnny. It is your turn to read. Where has your mind been today? We called on you three times." Johnny, of course, is subject to further ridicule, as he has no idea where to begin reading. While the class has been reading about the magical adventures of Harry Potter, Johnny has been wishing he too had magic powers or an invisibility cloak so that he could disappear—or at least get away from his abusive stepfather. Last night, Johnny feared for his life, for his baby brother's life, and for his mother's life when his father came home drunk and violent. Johnny's mind has been riveted on his horrific home life, but the teacher sees him only as "not paying attention."

"Authority Issues"

A student's difficulties in school may also be caused by an apparent lack of cooperation, or "an issue with authority." These situations too may have abuse- or neglect-related explanations. A student unwilling to dress down for gym may be avoiding classmates and gym teachers seeing otherwise hidden bruises or may feel shame or discomfort with his/her body following sexual abuse. Children "refusing" to wear their prescribed glasses may in fact not have glasses. Students who refuse to stay after school for an assigned detention may be hurrying home to protect younger siblings otherwise left alone or with a violent adult.

Teachers should be particularly attuned to sudden changes in performance or attitude. Is a child who was previously punctual, organized, and prepared now late, forgetting homework, and exhausted? Is a student who previously was a gregarious, active participant in class now silent and withdrawn?

Of course, academic problems are not always indicative of abuse, but the possibility of child maltreatment should be considered along with other possible explanations whenever the concerns are assessed (Tower, 1992).

"Overachieving"

Some children suffering from abuse, on the other hand, will excel academically. A focus on scholastics may be a means of coping (Nugent et al., 1998). Young children and adolescents may well choose to focus on their studies rather than the violence in their lives, even if only as a form of escapism. Perhaps when she is thinking about challenging algebra problems or writing a creative story, she is able to "escape" for a time and her mind is not on what her father did to her last night.

In other cases, children being abused may excel academically in an effort to please unpleasable, abusive parents. "If I get a 100 on this Social Studies exam, maybe Dad will stop yelling about what an embarrassing idiot I am." "Maybe if I make the honor roll, I won't be beaten when it's report card time." Perfectionistic attitudes and/or test anxiety may develop in such cases as these, but the children may do well academically.

Children like these, who have learned to work hard trying desperately to please their parents, may also be trying hard to please teachers as well. These students may be exceptionally conscientious, hypersensitive to any potential criticism, and may be overly concerned about meeting and exceeding every teacher expectation. While some of these students may be afraid of teachers, other students enjoy their relationships with teachers, as this may be their first experience with a safe, consistent, nurturing adult. These students may be observed to be staying around school as much as possible. For them, it offers a haven from the abuse and the one place to receive positive attention (Tower, 1992).

Thus, whether as an escape mechanism, or motivated by fear of parents or teachers, many children who are being abused do well in school. Thus, high-achieving students should not be assumed to be abuse free. School personnel should look beyond mere good grades to any extreme patterns of overexacting perfectionism, reluctance to leave school to go home, and other *possible* indicators of abuse.

Social/Emotional Behavioral Indicators

School personnel should also be alert to social and emotional indicators. As discussed in Chapter 1, children who are abused may externalize or internalize their distress. In some cases school professionals may notice a constellation of symptoms indicative of posttraumatic stress disorder (PTSD).

Those who externalize their distress may be observed as the school bullies, frequently responding to conflicts or social difficulty with aggression. This may be, in part, because many children who have been abused have developed a hostile attribution bias (Dodge, Pettit, Bates, & Valente, 1995). This "the-world-is-out-to get-me" attitude is obvious as these students interact with teachers and classmates, assuming they have to "fight back" even in the face of what would be considered by their peers as neutral or accidental situations. In addition to assuming hostile intent on the part of others, students who are aggressive may also have cognitive distortions regarding the legitimacy of aggression and retaliation, and immunity from consequences (Feindler, 1991). Given the histories of many of these children, this type of social information processing is understandable. The world has been "out to get them," and it is not a surprise that some would feel the need to "fight back." Garbarino (2000) describes this phenomenon, noting that children are "junior social anthropologists" who carefully observe how the world of human relationships works. Imagine the mental notes of an abused child: "Oh, I see, when people get mad, they get violent. And when you get violent, it is best to get violent with those most vulnerable. That way, you get away with it, because the person can't fight back and is too afraid to tell anyone."

Once school personnel know that a child has been abused, it may not be difficult for them to understand that externalizing symptoms might follow. However, it is important that the reasoning work in the opposite direction as well, that is, externalizing symptoms should raise the abuse question for school professionals. Diagnoses of behavior disordered, oppositional defiant disorder (ODD) or ADHD should not dissuade professionals from considering abuse. In fact, these diagnoses should encourage the question. That is not to say that all children with externalizing symptoms have been abused, but, as one study concluded, "Our findings suggest that many of the tens of thousands of children with disruptive behavior disorders may have been exposed to traumatic maltreatment and may experience undetected PTSD symptoms" (Ford et al., 2000, p. 214). While certainly most children with ADHD have not been maltreated, a sizable minority have. For children with ODD diagnoses, the rates of maltreatment are much higher—as high as 75% (Ford et al., 2000).

While some students who have been abused act out, others are excessively passive withdrawn, or uncommunicative. Anxiety and depression are among the most common postabuse symptoms. Again, consider the mental notes of some children who have experienced abuse: "The world is dangerous. Don't expect much good. Even those who are supposed to protect you may hurt you. Just lay low and you might avoid some of the bad." School personnel should be reminded to notice not only the difficult, acting out, or overtly disturbed students but also the particularly uncommunicative children, who are little trouble to their teachers but may be seriously depressed or anxious due to abuse, neglect, or some other difficult home situation (Fewster & Bagley, 1986).

School personnel may notice that, beyond being shy or introverted, some students develop posttraumatic abuse symptoms, becoming excessively fearful, or hypervigilant. They may seem afraid of teachers or coaches or "jumpy" when someone gestures in their direction. They may seem guarded, as if protecting secrets, afraid to let anyone get close. Social difficulties, perhaps related to externalizing or internalizing and/or other abuse-related symptomatology, are common. Children who are abused frequently have trouble being accepted by classmates. They may appear bizarre to other children, as some may occasionally "space out" during dissociative episodes.

Another abuse-specific symptom constellation that may be observed at school is sexual behavior problems. Many students who have been sexually abused have reactive behaviors in which their abuse, confusion, and pairing of sexuality and anger or sexuality and anxiety may be acted out. For example, a young girl was reported by her teacher to repeatedly masturbate against the corner of her desk each day during class. Other students may use bathroom breaks or find hidden places on the playground (e.g., behind bushes, in enclosed slides) to engage in, coerce, or force other children into sexual activity. It is important that school personnel be familiar with developmentally appropriate sexual behavior (see Table 2.2) so they may distinguish it from that which is problematic. When sexualized behavior involves others, professionals should be aware of the factors used in determining whether the behavior is experimentation or, rather, exploitation (see Table 2.3).

Sexual behavior problems, compared to more general symptoms of childhood distress (e.g., nightmares, anxiety, etc.), have more discriminative value (Yuille, Tymofievich, & Marxen, 1995). That is, they are more uniquely tied to abuse. However, it is important to note that children who exhibit sexual behavior problems have not always been directly sexually abused. Many times they are victims of other forms of maltreatment, or of no maltreatment at all. For example, consider a boy who is physically abused and

TABLE 2.2. Developmentally Appropriate Sexual Behaviors of Children

Early childhood

- Awareness of sexual body parts
- Curiosity about sexual body parts, evidenced by putting objects or fingers into genitals or rectum or asking questions about body parts or where babies come from
- Interest in showing and viewing private parts
- Random and sporadic self-exploration of body parts and genitalia, including masturbation (common times include when diapers are being changed, when going to sleep, when excited or afraid)
- Interest in bathroom functions
- Finds use of bathroom language or slang words for body parts funny
- May mimic obscene language of older children or adults but does not understand the meaning of the words
- Social games like imitation of marriage (e.g., kissing, hugging), playing doctor (e.g., examining others' bodies), or "show me yours, I'll show you mine"

Middle to late childhood

- Shows more modesty by needing privacy when changing clothes or going to the bathroom
- Curiosity about sex organs and bodily functions
- Masturbation occurs infrequently and in private
- Talks about sex or having babies with friends
- Uses more secrecy when talking about sexual matters, telling "dirty" jokes, or looking at nude pictures or watching erotic television programs or movies
- May engage in mutual touching or kissing with same-age peers or imitate sexual acts
- Plays games with opposite-sex peers related to sex (e.g., spin the bottle, kiss tag)
- Onset of puberty—physical and hormonal changes

Adolescence

- Concern with appearance and body image
- Demands more privacy
- Masturbation continues in private
- Consensual sexual experimentation, including petting, oral sex, intercourse, or infrequent mutual masturbation with a peer

Note. Information for this table was obtained from the following sources: Horton (1996); James and Burch (1999); Johnson (1999); and Tharinger (1987).

TABLE 2.3. Factors to Consider in Assessing the Nature of Child Sexual Behavior

♦ *Power differences.* Differences may exist in terms of the age (usually greater than 3 years), size, strength, social status, or intellectual abilities of the children involved. The larger the discrepancy, the greater the cause for concern.

♦ *Affect of children when "caught" by adults.* Giggly embarrassment is typical of curious exploration, while more intense reactions of shame, fear, anxiety, or anger at being discovered may be indicative of acts that are not mutual or consensual.

♦ *Response to correction.* Children involved in curious exploration will typically respond to correction or redirection; however, children who compulsively and/or defiantly repeat the behaviors should trigger more concern, as these children may not be able to, or do not want to, stop.

♦ *Specific sexual behaviors involved.* Behaviors that occur infrequently and to satisfy curiosity are part of normal sexual development. However, adult-type sexual acts (e.g., intercourse, oral-genital contact) or those beyond one's developmental level are more deserving of concern.

♦ *Means to compliance.* One clear sign that sexual behavior is problematic is when force, coercion, or threats have been used to gain compliance or maintain secrecy.

♦ *How the sexual behavior fits into the rest of the child's life.* If sexual behavior comes in and out of focus for a child and remains a small part of his/her life, it would be considered part of normal sexual development. On the other hand, if a child becomes so preoccupied with sexuality that it is interfering with or replacing appropriate activities or interests, then there is greater cause for concern.

Note. Information for this table was obtained from the following sources: Berliner and Rawlings (1991); Gil and Johnson (1993); Horton (1996); Johnson (1999); and Johnson and Friend (1995).

neglected. As part of the neglectful pattern, he is left unsupervised and able to have access to pornography. A child such as this may have the hurt and anger related to the maltreatment as well as the sexual knowledge needed to act out his distress in sexually aggressive ways. School personnel do not have to understand the precise etiology to be able to identify that a child may be being maltreated in some way.

Adolescents, too, may have sexual concerns and consequent sexual behavior problems. Often teens with an abuse history will tend toward one extreme or the other. They might "act out" sexually, having frequent, unprotected sex with multiple casual partners, or they may be fearful of the very thought of ever having sexual contact. If they have been abused by same-sex offenders (as is the case for many males), they may have concerns about what this means for their own sexual orientation. Again, they may be tempted to prove "just how heterosexual they are" by having many female sexual partners, or may experiment with same-sex partners, or may avoid sexual contact altogether.

Children who are neglected may also display behaviors specific to their maltreatment. They may be caught stealing or hoarding food. They may appear tired, listless, or sleepy. They might not have their required school materials. Once neglect is considered as a possible explanation, the behavior pattern makes greater sense. Absent any aspect of neglect, the student might seem simply dishonest, lazy, or disorganized.

Physical Indicators

Certainly children may be injured in a variety of nonabusive situations and circumstances; however, certain patterns should raise additional questions. For example, school personnel should take note when students have numerous bruises at various stage of healing (red, blue, black-purple, green tint dark, to pale green, to yellow) or when they wear makeup or inappropriate clothes (e.g., long sleeves in warm weather) to hide injuries (Tower, 1992). Burns (particularly those caused by cigarettes, irons, or hot water) should obviously raise serious questions. Welts (such as those that look like they were left from electrical cords, hangers, or belts), abdominal pain, swelling, tenderness, vomiting (possibly from blows to the stomach), or swelling in the head and dizziness (possibly from blows to the head or being thrown against a wall) should raise grave concern among school personnel (Tower, 1987, 1992).

Sexual abuse, in the vast majority of cases, leaves no physical effects (Lamb, 1994). Even when there is physical evidence of sexual abuse, it is typically hidden from school personnel. Occasionally there may be indicators, such as excessive vaginal scratching (due to discomfort caused by an infection or sexually transmitted disease) or, in rare extreme cases, a markedly different walk (due to genital tearing). Pregnancies on occasion are also indicators. In general, however, there are few, if any, obvious physical signs for school personnel to observe.

Neglect may have its own physical indicators that may be common at school, including poor hygiene (e.g., unlaundered clothes, frequent lice), hunger (as evidenced by stealing or hoarding food), and physical exhaustion (e.g., falling asleep in class) (Tower, 1992).

Parental Factors

Many abusive parents are charming and socially skilled in their interactions with adults, including school personnel. For example, David Pelzer, a survivor of horrific, tortuous child abuse, described his abusive mother as a "nice woman," active PTA member, and community "pillar"—whom nobody could believe would harm him (1995). Unfortunately, even seemingly "nice people" may be abusing their children. While interactions with parents may prove deceiving, sometimes there are warning signals. When told about the school's concerns regarding their children's behavior problems or distress, some abusive parents may tend to minimize or deny the problems. Others may blame, belittle, or demonize their child. If parents can find nothing good, positive, or attractive about their child, school personnel should take note (Tower, 1992). If they seem to be unaware of developmentally appropriate expectations and/or lack parenting skills, they will be more at risk for using abusive techniques. When parents seem unconcerned about their children, fail to make or keep appointments, or refuse to discuss problems, this could be a serious concern (Tower, 1992). If parents abuse drugs and/or alcohol, behave in bizarre or irrational ways, have a history of marital violence, or are in constant economic straits, the risks are even greater. Reports of "babysitting" by young children or indications of parent–child role reversal (e.g., a young child repeatedly "taking care of Mommy") may be cause for concern. Finally, if families have no "lifeline" or evidence of support (or sense of community), children are at greater risk (Tower, 1992).

Again, with most of these possible indicators, school personnel should be careful to not conclude too quickly that there is reason to suspect abuse or neglect. Patterns should be considered as many of the symptoms do not in and of themselves reliably predict maltreatment. Few indicators are, however, as reliable as a child's disclosure.

CHILD INTERVIEWS AND DISCLOSURES

Often, a school professional may have concerns regarding possible child maltreatment based on observed physical, emotional, or behavioral indicators but may need additional information. In other cases, a child may make a direct disclosure regarding abuse to someone at school. In either of these situations, a school professional may need to interview the child further to gain enough information to make a report (Brassard et al., 1983). Before moving to specific interview suggestions, two relevant subjects should be considered, namely, the disclosure process and the reliability of children's reports.

Disclosure Literature

On the surface, disclosure clearly seems like a good idea for a number of reasons. First, there is some intrinsic benefit in telling the secret—"getting it off one's chest," so to speak. Second, disclosure allows for potential intervention to stop the abuse. Finally, disclosure increases the likelihood that a child will get treatment and learn, among other things, that the abuse is not his/her fault (Devoe & Faller, 1999).

A naive assumption might be that most children who are abused will tell someone immediately. Clearly, however, this is not the case. In the case of sexual abuse, for example, as few as one-third of victims may tell someone at the time of the abuse (Arata, 1998). Many wait years, even decades, to tell, and some never tell at all.

A number of variables may influence a child's disclosure decision. One important variable is the nature and severity of the abuse. While one might assume that those with "minor" abuse experiences are the ones who are not reporting (perhaps because they do not see the need), this is not the case. In fact, those least likely to disclose may be those with the most severe abuse. Arata (1998) found that survivors of sexual abuse with the more invasive, longer-lasting experiences and those perpetrated by relatives were least likely to disclose. It appears that, if a child does not disclose soon after the initial contact, he/she may be more reluctant to disclose as the abuse goes on. "Perhaps the decrease in disclosure results from children's beliefs that if they did not tell after the first incident, they will be blamed for letting it continue" (Arata, 1998, p. 69).

Children's willingness or ability to disclose is dependent on a number of variables, including age, maternal support, threat or coercion, offender–victim relationship, severity of the abuse, and posttraumatic stress (Devoe & Faller, 1999). Offenders' threats may be a particularly powerful influence in the delay of a disclosure. Perpetrators may threaten that the child will get in trouble, or even be put in jail, if he/she tells. Offenders may tell the child it will be "all their fault" if people find out, the family is broken up, or Mommy is upset. Some offenders even make violent threats, promising to kill themselves, the child, other family members, or a much-loved family pet if the child tells anyone. Thus, clearly it is understandable why many children will, at least initially, deny that they are being abused. Simply put, "Denial has been identified as a frequent response when the child is feeling too threatened, frightened, or insecure to acknowledge the abuse" (Sorenson & Snow, 1991, p. 4).

Additionally, even those who do disclose often do so accidentally or unintentionally. This is especially the case with young children. Their sexual behavior or language gives them away. The "secret" that they told a peer is shared with an adult. Or, in some cases, it is simply determined that an alleged or convicted offender (in legal trouble for other cases) had extensive contact with this child (Sorensen & Snow, 1991).

Those who do disclose intentionally often do so after they have been prompted in some way. Many disclose after an educational program at school, with the encouragement of peers, just after the offender has moved away, or because something else in the immediate environment triggered the disclosure (Sorenson & Snow, 1991).

Disclosure Is a Process

Spontaneous disclosures in which a child suddenly tells someone his or her entire story are relatively rare. Much more frequently, disclosure is a gradual process (Devoe & Faller, 1999). Disclosure often unfolds and becomes more detailed over multiple interviews (Devoe & Faller, 1999). Children often go through a process of several steps (Sorenson & Snow, 1991).

- ◆ Denial
- ◆ Tentative disclosure
- ◆ Active disclosure
- ◆ Recantation
- ◆ Reaffirmation

This process is not always a positive experience. Disclosures, in many cases, are additionally traumatic events. Hindman (1999) coined the phrase "disclosure disasters" to describe disclosure reactions that, instead of being supportive, made things worse. Put simply, "The response to disclosure seemed to add trauma rather than assist in the healing process. The victim would have been better off to have never reported" (Hindman, 1999, p. 87).

Consider one disturbing case Hindman (1999) shares to illustrate the point:

> Karen is sexually abused by her brother for approximately three years. As Karen becomes more aware of the inappropriateness of her brother's sexual behavior, she finally reports to her mother. Karen's mother becomes extremely upset, screaming at her, and eventually sends Karen to her room. Karen's mother forbids Karen to eat dinner with the rest of the family. Finally, Karen is brought into the living room, and her father proceeds to beat Karen's brother unmercifully. Karen reports being barely able to recognize her brother when the beating concluded. Her mother sobs, but does not comfort Karen in any way. Bleeding and nearly unrecognizable, Karen's brother is forced to apologize on bended knee for his transgression. That same evening Karen lies in bed and listens to her brother crying. Suddenly, her father enters the room and quietly rapes Karen. (p. 87)

In this disturbing case, as in all 188 of the severely traumatized cases in Hindman's sample who made a disclosure, the response to the disclosure was disastrous.

In another case of a disastrous postreport response, Hindman tells of three sixth-grade boys who were sexually abused by a school teacher. The school faculty found it impossible to believe that the teacher could have done such a thing. Rather than supporting the boys, or even remaining neutral, teachers and fellow students put intense pressure on the boys to recant and "admit their lies." The school created a situation in which the boys became very fearful. The school openly held a car wash and bake sale to raise money for the teacher's defense. While the boys won a civil court case in the matter, Hindman points out they did not really win. Two of the boys dropped out of school, and one committed suicide. The abuse had been bad enough, but the school's response had added to the trauma.

Other studies have confirmed that victims with adverse responses to disclosure have higher levels of distress, psychopathology, and dissociation (Arata, 1998; Everill & Waller, 1995; Roesler, 1994). Given these negative experiences, it is not surprising that many adult survivors report regretting their decision to disclose. Schools should strive to avoid contributing to any "disclosure disasters." School professionals should always do what they can to handle disclosures in such a way that victims will not later regret their decisions. Thus, the practical suggestions provided toward the end of this chapter are especially important.

THE RELIABILITY OF CHILD REPORTERS

In addition to the literature regarding disclosures, research regarding children's reliability as reporters is important to consider. Some may wonder whether you can trust the accuracy of a child's story. Did the child just make it up to get attention? There are three major concerns that arise in this literature. First, it is a very new field. Second, much of what has been written is less than objective. Third, laboratory research methods may not reflect actual clinical experience.

A New Field

Faller (1996) points out that, while there is a growing knowledge base, the field is new and there are many unknowns. "In the context of child protection intervention in North America, the idea of asking children what happened when they may have been maltreated is a fairly novel concept" (Faller, 1996, p. 83). "Until recently there was little scientific data regarding children's eyewitness testimony" (Saywitz & Goodman, 1996, p. 297). The field has come a long way in the past two decades; however, there are still unanswered questions (Faller, 1996).

In addition to the novelty of the field, the emotionally charged nature of the discussion may be difficult for practitoners to sort out. "Irresponsible claims such as 'children never lie' about being sexually abused" and, conversely, "the vast majority of children who profess sexual abuse in the context of custody litigation are 'fabricators' are not supported by empirical research and serve to inflame rather than clarify the complexities of this subject"

(Reed, 1994, p. 127). "Such polarization, fueled by strong emotions, some-times results in extreme bias, exaggerated claims, and an atmosphere of an-tagonism in an area where objectivity, a balanced perspective, and coopera-tion among professionals are so crucial" (Reed, 1996, p. 106).

Research Methods

The methodology of the rather limited research studies in this area rarely in-volves actual cases of child abuse victims. While it is understandable that eth-ical limitations, funding issues, and other obstacles exist to including abuse victims, it is difficult to know how closely lab analogs match "the real world" (Faller, 1996). Unfortunately, it is likely that, even with good intentions and careful laboratory controls, even "the best experimental research has limited applicability to the dynamic, complex, and delicate process of forensically in-terviewing suspected child abuse victims" (Reed, 1996, p. 106).

Research regarding children's ability to report accurately and not be in-fluenced by suggestible and misleading techniques has typically examined only one direction. These are not unidimensional phenomena, that is, excess-es may occur on either side of the question. While much concern has been raised about children being led to make false allegations, "it is equally true that abused children can be misled to minimize or to completely deny abuse that they have suffered" (Reed, 1996, p. 107).

Suggestibility

In spite of these limitations, there are some important findings to consider in areas regarding children's abuse reporting. One major concern in this area of suggestibility—which may be defined as the degree to which one's "memo-ry" and/or "recounting" of an event is influenced by suggested information or misinformation—is that it could lead to inaccurate memories or inaccu-rate reporting (Reed, 1996, p. 106). In reviewing the literature, Reed (1996, pp. 107–113) draws the following conclusions for practitioners to consider:

- Suggestibility is not a "trait" that remains constant for an individual regardless of the circumstances.
- Preschool children tend to be more vulnerable to suggestion than do either school-aged children or adults.
- Certain types of questions, suggestions, and props are more likely to mislead some children under certain circumstances.
- Children are more likely to be misled when they do not understand what is expected of them.
- Both children and adults tend to be more easily misled when their memory for the event in question is weak.

- Children tend to be more suggestible when they perceive the interviewer to be authoritarian, unfriendly, or intimidating.
- Children tend to be more suggestible when they think the interviewer is knowledgeable about the event in question.

While child interviewing may be important in all forms of maltreatment, it may be most critical in sexual abuse cases. Physical abuse or neglect cases may have physical and/or medical evidence that can be used to determine what occurred, but in cases of sexual abuse there is rarely such evidence. Instead, there is typically a situation that occurred in secret that only two people know about: the offender (who is disinclined to admit what took place) and a child (Faller, 1996). "Thus, child interviewing, as a way of understanding maltreatment, derives from the virtual absence of other alternatives in reports of sexual abuse" (Faller, 1996, p. 84).

Improper and misleading interviewing techniques have been employed in some cases of suspected child maltreatment; however, the extent of the problem has not been studied empirically (Reed, 1996). "In light of the potentially grave consequences associated with arriving at erroneous conclusions in cases of suspected child maltreatment, it is incumbent on all professionals involved in investigation and decision making to be guided by the most reliable information available" (Reed, 1996, p. 106).

Based on the findings from the research and clinical literature, Reed (1996) and others have suggested some specific strategies in the four areas of interview setting, interview characteristics, clarifying expectations, and questioning strategies. Many of the suggestions are applicable even to school professionals doing brief interviews to determine the possible necessity of a child abuse report. School professionals should carefully consider aspects of interviewing so that a legally defensible disclosure may be obtained and, more importantly, so they can facilitate truth seeking.

Whether following up on indicators of abuse (Brassard et al., 1983) or responding to a child's disclosure (Johnson, 1989), the school psychologist or other professional should be careful to conduct a clinically sensitive, yet legally defensible, nonleading interview. The most important aspect of a child interview may be a warm, caring, nonjudgmental style. Although variations in individual style are acceptable (Johnson, 1989), some key points are important for all to consider.

Interview Setting

Interviews relating to suspected child maltreatment, even the brief "should-we-make-a-call-to-Child-Protection?" type of interviews done at school, should be conducted in a private setting. Given the possible shame, embarrassment, and confusion that a victim of abuse may already be experiencing, school personnel must be especially sensitive to issues of privacy. While practical constraints may exist, it is imperative that the school professional find an appropriately private location rather than using a hallway or corner of a classroom where other students or school personnel may overhear the conversation. A child victim may be more likely to deny the abuse if he/she fears others may be listening to the conversation (Horton, 1995).

The child being questioned should feel reasonably comfortable. The environment should be informal and free from distracting commotion or props (Reed, 1996). There has been a movement in the child protection field to avoid interviewing children in police stations, or at least to modify the environment. In earlier years, children might have ended up sitting at a regular police investigator's desk, facing a uniformed officer—perhaps one even carrying a gun. Clearly this environment was inconsistent with the messages intended for victims, namely, "you are not in trouble" or "it's OK—just tell me what happened." Modified police department offices—many with nonuniformed, nonarmed officers, and even special child advocacy centers—are replacing the old context. Similar considerations should be made at school. While the principal's office may be available, using this room may send an unintentional message such as "you're in trouble—be careful what you say."

Interviewer Characteristics

A typical school scenario might involve a teacher who "just thinks something is not right" about Susie's behavior following a recent stay with her grandparents. The teacher, however, feels uncomfortable asking Susie about any details. The teacher asks the school psychologist or the school social worker for help. Who should talk to Susie? Often the issue of gender is considered first; however, this may not be as important as one might think. The key consideration may be the ability to be friendly and maintain a rapport with the child (Reed, 1996). A calm, informal tone should be maintained throughout the interview. Rather than immediately starting to take notes and engage in a full-scale interrogation, the school professional should more informally converse with the child, starting with more general nonthreatening subjects, and leading up to topics related to the suspected abuse. Once the child begins discussing the abuse, it is important that the school professional remain attentive yet calm. The display of extreme disgust, horror, or shock might alarm the child and shut down further disclosure. Often a child will tell about a limited aspect of the abuse experience initially, as if to test the interviewer. If the child concludes that the interviewer "can't handle it," he/she may not go on to tell what else happened. Basic good listening skills and child-oriented communication abilities are imperative throughout the interview. The educator should listen carefully to what the child is saying while at the same time taking close note of any nonverbal communication clues.

One of the most important aspects of the interviewer's attitude and behavior is the need to approach the interview with an open mind. Often it is difficult not to approach the child with a predetermined notion that "it couldn't be." This may be particularly difficult if the child is speaking about a member of the school faculty or staff (Hindman, 1999) or a much loved parent who is active in the school community (Pelzer, 1995).

The interviewer should work to use developmentally appropriate language and concepts, noticing and using the child's words. As with any sensitive clinical work, the school professional should listen and validate how the child feels rather than guessing or telling him/her how he/she must feel. Given the wide variety of abuse experiences children have suffered and the various feeling stages that each child may go through, one really cannot assume what the child feels. Thus, comments such as "I'm sure you feel guilty, but you shouldn't" or "I know you're angry—you have a right to be," while well intentioned perhaps, are generally not helpful (Horton, 1995).

Clarifying Expectations

First, the school professional must be clear about the limits to confidentiality. Sometimes, before answering any questions about abuse, children may attempt to get school professionals to make promises of absolute confidentiality (e.g., "If I tell you something very, very secret, will you promise not to tell?"). Instead of naively agreeing, one must be clear with a child (in developmentally appropriate terms) about the limits to confidentiality, clarifying that if a child is being hurt, that is not a good secret to keep (Horton, 1995). While it is certainly possible that an honest discussion regarding confidentiality at the outset may prevent a child from disclosing abuse at that time, the child may ultimately appreciate the interviewer's honesty, realize that this is a person who can be trusted, and make a more complete disclosure later.

Many of the specific suggestions about clarifying expectations of the interviewee that have been made in the literature are more applicable to CPS workers or others conducting forensic interviews (see Reed, 1996, for further discussion); however, some of the suggestions do apply to school-based practice. For example, it is a good idea to clarify to the child that the interviewer is uninformed. Children, particularly young children, have been found to be less reliable reporters if they believe that the person asking questions already knows what happened. For example, "I wasn't in your classroom the day that substitute, Mr. Jones, was there. So, I don't know what happened. Tell me about it." An additional applicable suggestion is encouraging children to be honest, including sharing their confusion, not knowing an answer, or not wanting to talk about it (Reed, 1996).

Questioning Strategies

Perhaps most of the research and related suggestions regarding disclosures focuses on the questioning strategies used during the interview. Developmentally appropriate language should certainly be used across all strategies (Reed, 1996).

In general, it is important not to have the child go through repetitive interviews, which may inadvertently suggest to a child that he/she is not answering correctly or that people are waiting for a different answer. This should be noted as a particular risk at school. It is not difficult to imagine a scenario in which a child begins to disclose abuse to a teacher. The teacher, feeling "out of her league," may take the child to speak with the principal. The principal may ask the child a few questions but then, not sure how to proceed, may call for the school psychologist to join the conversation. At this point, the child has already been interviewed three times. This has all occurred before CPS has even been contacted. Child protection workers will likely have their own interview (or interviews). Additionally, in many cases, the police, the State's attorney, and other attorneys may interview the child. Certainly, the "system" is making efforts to reduce the number of interviews via child advocacy centers, one-way mirrors, and joint interviews; however, repeated interviews are often still the norm. The school should not increase this list. Once there is enough information to reasonably suspect abuse, the interviewing should stop. There is no need to get corroboration from three or four school professionals that, in fact, this is reportable. It should be noted that, while it is bad practice to have a child face repeated formal interviews at school, that does not mean that it is not a good idea for someone close to the child (e.g., a teacher) to have ongoing dialogue with the child. Disclosure is typically a drawn-out process (Sorenson & Snow, 1991) in which the child may initially tell the teacher just a small portion, then a little more, then take it back, and later tell the full story.

Again, school professionals are reminded that they need not, and must not, try to function in the role of child abuse investigator. However, there are still situations in which some questioning of children is necessary before the appropriate professionals can determine whether they suspect abuse and must make a report. Thus, it is helpful for school practitioners to be aware of the available information regarding various questioning techniques.

Question types can be considered on a continuum, from open-ended/free-recall strategies on one extreme to highly leading questions on the other extreme. In between are focused and specific questioning techniques. Each type of question has its own advantages and disadvantages, and those interviewing children, including those in school settings, should select their questions carefully, being aware of these considerations.

Open-Ended Questions

Open-ended questions are those without direction or limitation from the questioner. A child's free recall in response to an open-ended question is thought to be the most accurate form of memory report (Reed, 1996; Saywitz & Goodman, 1996). Inquiries such as "what happened?" or "tell me what has been going on" suggest no preconceived direction or even topic from the person conducting the interview. Thus, responses are assumed to come from the child's own mind and hopefully the child's own experience (Reed, 1996). On the surface, one would think that given this tendency, only open-ended questions should be asked.

Unfortunately, open-ended questions have their disadvantages as well. Without some direction, children may not discuss the "right thing," that is, the issues regarding the possible abuse (Lamb, 1994; Reed, 1996; Saywitz & Goodman, 1996). They may describe an event that actually occurred but is of no interest to the interviewer (Saywitz & Goodman, 1996). For example, to the question "what has been happening in your life?" a child may tell in some detail about recent soccer games, school grades, or social events. Many children, particularly very young children, will not respond at all to open-ended questions, or they will simply answer "nothing." Thus, this type of question often generates the least information. In sum, open-ended questions often result in errors of omission or false negatives (Reed, 1996). Their use, therefore, is important but may not be enough.

Leading Questions

On the opposite end of the continuum, highly leading questions are those that "suggest new information and tempt, pressure, or coerce a child to agree with suggested information" (Reed, 1996, p. 109). For example, "Your father touched your privates, didn't he?" or "I'm sure your mother didn't give you that bruise on purpose. It was an accident, wasn't it?" Children may answer these questions; however, especially very young children may be inaccurate in their responses and may feel compelled to answer as they suspect that the interviewer wants them to answer. For these reasons, such questions are the "riskiest" (Reed, 1996) and should typically be avoided, especially in school settings.

Focused or Direct Questions

Between the two ends of the continuum are focused or specific questions. Focused questions are those that "may introduce a new topic but do not combine the identity of the 'actor' with a potentially abusive 'action'" (Reed, 1996, p. 109). For example, a school practitioner might say, "I understand you have been visiting at your Dad's house. How are the visits going? Tell me what you like about the visits. Is there anything that you don't like? " This form of questioning has received mixed reviews. While some critics fear that such questions are dangerously suggestive, many believe they may be necessary to elicit reliable information about possible abuse (Reed, 1996). While there has been a paucity of empirical research regarding these types of question, there is general agreement that they are acceptable and even necessary to elicit information from children (Lamb, 1994; Reed, 1996). They seem to help trigger reports that would otherwise not be available.

Direct questions have been the subject of more empirical investigation. These questions, because they *do* combine the identity of the actor with some potentially abusive action, are somewhat more suggestive (Reed, 1996). One example might be "Did that substitute teacher ever touch your private parts?" While there are concerns about the increased level of suggestibility, empirical evidence has documented that such questions may be necessary and may not result in as many false reports as one might think. For example, in a study involving interviews of 72 children following a routine medical exam, the vast majority (78% and 89%) of children failed to reveal vaginal and/or anal touching, respectively, in response to open-ended questions asking them to "tell everything you remember about your visit to the doctor's office." When asked more directly about vaginal and anal touching, only 14% and 21%, respectively, failed to reveal the touching, and there were very few "false reports." Only three answered "yes" incorrectly to the direct questions about vaginal or anal touching, and two of the three did not elaborate. Thus, for skilled forensic interviewers (who know how to carefully follow up and check for a child's ability to elaborate), there may be some legitimate use of these direct questions. *However, the risks may outweigh the benefits for school personnel.*

In general, then, school-based interviews should begin with open-ended questions that allow a child the opportunity to freely recall what he/she would like to report. If this does not result in a discussion of the abuse-related subject, more focused questioning may be used in follow-up. Highly leading questions should certainly not be used, and even direct questions should be avoided by school-related professionals.

Follow-Up with the Child

At the conclusion of the interview, it is important for the school psychologist to explain, as much as possible, what will happen next. For example, if the child has disclosed abuse, the school professional should inform the child that the abuse will be reported and what he/she might expect to happen. While the practitioner clearly will not be able to say definitively how CPS will proceed, a good working relationship with such agencies allows school-based professionals to have some idea of the likely response for various types of abuse reports. The school professional might be able to tell an adolescent who has suffered mild physical abuse, "A social worker may call your parents and ask what has been going on or to suggest a counselor." On the other hand, a school psychologist might warn a young sexual abuse victim, "The police may come to school to talk to you. That does not mean you are in trouble. They will be trying to help you." Another aspect of informing the child about what they can anticipate next is to be clear with the child about what they can expect from the school practitioner. It is important to be honest with oneself and with the child. As well-intentioned, caring people who are deeply concerned about child victims, some professionals may be tempted to volunteer for more than they can really do. A realistic explanation of "I'll be checking in with you every week or so, and you can ask your teacher to contact me in an emergency" may be more honest than "I'll stick with you through this whole thing. I'll go to court. I'll be with you wherever you go, whatever you need." Since most school practitioners are overburdened with multiple demands, clear boundaries are better for everyone concerned.

Given the importance and complexity of this work, whenever possible, school personnel should allow trained personnel from an abuse agency to handle the interviews (Brassard et al., 1983). School professionals should conduct interviews only to gain information to make the report, which will then involve abuse experts.

Keeping in mind that children rarely lie about abuse, and that it is important only to get enough information to make a report since others will do a more investigative interview, school practitioners should generally assume that the voluntarily self-reporting child is telling the truth and act accordingly. Direct or subtle messages of disbelief may squelch the child's further disclosure. Instead, the child should be reassured that telling someone was the right thing to do.

Documentation

When the interview is completed, the interviewer should document the conversation in as much detail as possible, accurately and adequately recording relevant questions and responses. Without being obtrusive or overly formal, some professionals prefer to jot brief notes during the interview, including key phrases used by the child, and fill in extra details after the interview. Others, depending on state and district regulations, tape record the interview and take notes while listening to the tape. The child should be informed accordingly.

False Allegations

While it may be a slight exaggeration to say that "children *never* lie about abuse," researchers believe that only a very small percentage (less than 10%) of allegations made by children are false (Everson & Boat, 1989; Jones & McGraw, 1987; Yuille et al., 1995). The few children who do make false allegations have frequently been asked by an adult to do so. Those arising solely from children, then, are extremely rare. School professionals may be tempted to dismiss allegations made by children who are generally manipulative, out of control, or bizarre; however, it must be kept in mind that these very characteristics may actually be symptoms of abuse.

"False Memory Syndrome" and Repression

An extensive discussion of the "false memory syndrome" debate is beyond the scope of this text; however, it is important that school personnel have some basic understanding of these issues so that judgment is not clouded in responding to abuse issues. This matters for two reasons. First, those who hear through the media about "false memory syndrome" as a pervasive phenomenon may begin to question incidence and prevalence rates, such as those discussed earlier in Chapter 1. Second, school personnel may be confronted with situations in which children or adolescents report incidents of abuse from some years back.

First and foremost, it is important to notice that two separate questions have been confused in much of the public and even professional discussions. One question is "Can false memories be planted in situations such as therapy?" This, however, is a separate question from "Can accurate memories be repressed (or forgotten) and later recalled?" Unfortunately, too often in this emotionally charged debate, it has been suggested that if the answer to the first question is "yes," then the answer to the second one must necessarily be "no."

Research on each of these questions must be considered separately. Memory researchers (e.g., Loftus & Yapko, 1995) have pointed out that "memory is suggestible" and that therapists might inadvertently be "planting memories" in their clients' minds. Laboratory research has confirmed that a sizable proportion of people (approximately 25%) can be led to recall events that may have been a false memory (e.g., being lost in a mall). It appears, however, that it is more difficult to create false memories of a more personal nature (e.g., childhood enemas) (Pezdek & Hodge, 1999). So, can memories be suggested? It appears that, at least at some level, the answer is "yes."

The answer to the second question, however, also appears to be "yes." Memories can be repressed or forgotten and later recalled. Briere and Conte (1993) interviewed 450 women and men with histories of sexual abuse, and over 50% acknowledged a period of partial to total amnesia for the abuse. In another remarkable study, this one on medically documented cases of sexual abuse, Williams (1994) found that 38% of women, interviewed years later, had no memory of their childhood sexual abuse and related emergency room visits.

So, what are the implications of these findings for school practitioners? First, memories of abuse should never be suggested to a student because he or she "seems like" an abuse victim. Second, however, if students themselves report previously forgotten memories of abuse, these disclosures should be taken as seriously as any others.

CONCLUSION

School personnel have been identified as key respondents to child maltreatment largely because they constitute society's primary out-of-home contact with children (home is where most abuse occurs). This environment ideally provides opportunities to identify abused children and begin initial steps in providing for their protection and securing needed intervention. To use this opportunity properly, school health practitioners must have realistic attitudes, be able to identify possible indicators, and be prepared to respond sensitively and effectively to student disclosures.

◆◆◆

Reporting Suspected
Child Maltreatment

◆

Once the question of child abuse has been raised, through child disclosures and/or professional observations of indicators, the decision whether to make a report must be considered. "Because the impact of filing a report of alleged child maltreatment can be great, it is not surprising that the decision to file is a difficult one for many mandated reporters" (Levine et al., 1995, p. 45). This chapter will address the rationales, logistics, and dilemmas of reporting suspected child maltreatment.

THE RATIONALE FOR REPORTING

Legal, ethical, and moral considerations require that school personnel report suspected child abuse and neglect.

Legal Considerations

Reporting laws are a relatively recent phenomenon. Initial legislative efforts began after Kempe's landmark "Battered Child Syndrome" address in 1962. The 1974 Child Abuse Prevention and Treatment Act (Public Law 93-247) provided federal funds to states with specific laws and procedures regarding reporting and investigating child abuse and neglect. Initially laws required only that physicians report suspected child maltreatment. By the 1980s, however, states were including many other professional groups, in particular mental health and school personnel (Zellman & Faller, 1996).

Currently each state has an *Abused and Neglected Child Act* that requires a wide range of professionals (in some states, all citizens) to report suspected child maltreatment (Illinois Department of Child and Family Services [ID-CFS], 1998). Since there is some variability regarding reporting specifics, such as which agency should be contacted and time frames of written and oral reports, it is critical that school professionals be familiar with the laws in their state.

State laws, and in some cases manuals for mandated reporters, may be obtained by contacting child protection departments in each state. Additionally, they are available via the following website: *http://www.calib. com/nccanch/pubs/sag/mandatory.pdf*. The National Clearinghouse on Child Abuse and Neglect Information publication *Statutes at a Glance,* which can be found at this site, provides an overview of state laws. Other related publications are available from the clearinghouse at *http://www.calib. com/nccanch*. Additionally, the website *http://www.smith-lawfirm.com/ mandatory_reporting.htm* provides an overview and has links to each state's statutes.

While there is some variability among states, certain important aspects are consistent. School personnel are clearly named in each state as one of the professional groups of mandated reporters. Some state laws mention the general category only; others specifically name teachers, school psychologists, and principals. In either case, school professionals are all mandated reporters.

Mandated, by definition, is the opposite of voluntary, or optional. Mandated reporters, therefore, are *required by law* to report suspected child abuse and neglect. Failure to report is considered a class B misdemeanor as a negligent party, and fines may be associated with the offense (Brassard et al., 1983; IDCFS, 1998).

No state requires that school personnel have proof of abuse at the time of the report but rather only a "reason to suspect" (or the like) before a report is mandated. Thus, school personnel are warned not to wait until they have irrefutable evidence. Even when professionals are clear that they must make a call when they suspect abuse, there is still some lack of clarity about what constitutes abuse. For example, at what point does spanking cross over to "excessive corporal punishment" or "physical abuse"? How young is too young to be left alone? At what point is that neglect? When is a dirty house a health and safety concern? What is the difference between poverty and neglect (IDCFS, 1998)? A rule of thumb to consider when making such determinations is "Has the child been harmed or been at substantial risk of harm?" (IDCFS, 1998, p. 7).

Once you have decided that you have reasonable cause to believe abuse or neglect has occurred, then an immediate oral report typically must be made to the state CPS agency. Written follow-up may be required within a slightly longer time period (e.g., 48 hours). States generally have some sort of "good Samaritan" clause to protect mandated reporters. School personnel, therefore, have immunity from civil liability and/or criminal penalty when they do report maltreatment, provided the report is made in good faith (Brassard et al., 1983).

In sum, the law is quite clear that school personnel are required to report suspected child abuse and neglect. In fact, they may be considered legally negligent if they do not report their suspicions. Regardless of the outcome of the report and/or investigation, school personnel with honest reason for concern are legally protected from any civil or criminal penalties related to the report. Legally, the duty to report is quite clear.

Ethical Considerations

Beyond legal requirements, most school professionals have as a part of their professional ethical codes the mandate to act in the best interests of the students and to follow state laws. This would certainly include the ethical mandate to report suspected child abuse and neglect. Thus, to suspect but not report abuse would be in violation of professional ethics. Such a decision would put one at risk for ethical charges within the professional organization and, in some cases, at least, potentially jeopardize licensure or certification.

While reporting suspected child abuse and neglect seems consistent with professional ethics, numerous competing ethical standards do create dilemmas for the professional. For example, mental heath professional codes consistently mention confidentiality as a principal professional value. When one makes the decision to report, either to child protection or the police, suspicions or disclosures of abuse or neglect, the ideal principle of confidentiality is violated. Personal information is shared beyond the child client or family. Much has been written about the impact of such a decision on therapeutic relationships (see, for example, Levine et al., 1995). Distrust and/or a sense of betrayal often develops, and many clients will leave treatment after a report is made (Levine et al., 1995). These issues may also apply to relationships with school personnel. Families and child or adolescent clients may feel angry, violated, or betrayed by a professional they believed they could trust. Families may move away from the school or at least cancel their children's participation in any counseling relationships. Thus, this apparent conflict between competing ethical principles may create understandable dilemmas for professionals as they attempt to weigh confidentiality concerns against the potential abuse of children.

Pope and Vasquez (1991) have written about the conceptual basis for ethical principles. They note that trust, power, and caring are the grounds for most professional ethics. Thus, when struggling with a dilemma, the school professional should recognize that to act consistently with one principle might to a certain extent violate another. Professionals are encouraged to consider not simply specific ethical codes but also their intent. In order to act in way that is consistent with not just the "letter of the law," but the "spirit" of the ethical codes, one would ask questions such as the following:

> "This child has placed his/her *trust* in me. How can I act in his/her best interests?"
>
> "I have the *power* of privileged information. How will I use it for good?"
>
> "Given all that I understand may be happening in this child's life, what is the *caring* thing for me to do?"

Once professionals begin to consider the foundation for these ethical principles, they may begin to move toward the next rationale for reporting, the moral considerations.

Moral Considerations

Beyond what state law or professional ethical codes require, school professionals have a moral responsibility to report likely child abuse because of their personal commitment to the well-being of children (Tower, 1992). Put simply, as stated in an Illinois Department of Child and Family Services brochure, "Care enough to call." Without someone willing to make a report, children are denied the protection they need, at times, from severe abuse and imminent harm (Zellman & Faller, 1996). On a case-by-case basis, reports may protect children from severe physical injury or even death. Psychological suffering may be lessened and dysfunctional patterns interrupted. Families may get needed services. Pelzer (1995), a survivor of horrific abuse and now a prolific author and speaker, talks pointedly about the school personnel who had the courage to acknowledge and report his abuse, and those who did not.

Similar remarks are made in *Dear Teacher, If You Only Knew . . .* (Seryak, 1997) a compilation of poignant letters written by adults reflecting on their histories of child abuse and their experiences in school. Consider the following examples:

> "As I reflect on the teachers who may have realized something wasn't quite right or that abuse may have been occurring, I wish they had acted on what they might have suspected or even knew." (Annie, p. 18)

> "I don't blame you. How could you have known? But, if you had asked, it would have all come pouring out. The sex, the beating, the neglect—all of it! Please don't be afraid to ask!" (Erin, p. 61)

> "I finally got the courage to tell a teacher what was happening to me. Instead of believing me, the teacher wrote a letter to my parents. For punish-

ment . . . I was beaten more severely and taken out of school for good."
(Shirley, p. 103)

Such remarks by victims who survived with little support from the
schools should remind school professionals that beyond legal or even professional ethical rationales, there are moral reasons to report suspected abuse—
to protect the individual child, to prevent serious injury, and even to prevent
years of emotional suffering.

In addition to case-by-case decisions, which may literally be life-or-
death matters or at least life-changing decisions, professionals must consider
the moral basis for decisions as a group. Collectively, the accurate assessment
of incidence helps federal and state governments respond appropriately with
needed funds and policies (Zellman & Faller, 1996). Insufficient information
(based on lack of follow-through or blatant bureaucratic obstacles to reporting) may lead to insufficient funding and inappropriate policy decisions.
Thus, victims may be left without services they desperately need.

LOGISTICS OF REPORTING

To Whom Should a Report Be Made?

School professionals should consult their specific state laws to determine who
should be the recipient of their reports. However, in general, the following
guidelines apply.

Child Protective Services, in most states, is the appropriate recipient of
most child abuse reports. Illinois law, for example, stipulates which cases
should be reported to CPS (called the Department of Child and Family Services in that state; IDCFS, 1998). In regard to child victims 17 years old and
younger, the following categories of alleged perpetrators would be under
their purview:

- Parents
- Individuals living in the household
- Persons in an "official capacity or a position of trust" (e.g., teacher,
  health care professional, volunteer in a youth program)
- Persons responsible for the welfare of the child (e.g., babysitter, day
  care worker)

In most states some sort of 24-hour "hotline" is available so that reports
can be made to CPS immediately. While the alleged-perpetrator categories
above certainly would encompass many of the reports that school personnel
would be making, not all situations are included. For example, if a child is
suspected of having been abused by a neighbor who was not also babysitting

the child, this may not be a CPS matter. Also, in the rare event of an alleged stranger abusing a child, this too would be beyond CPS's jurisdiction. However, this does not mean that these situations should go unreported but rather they should be referred to the police. Additionally, cases involving older adolescents (in Illinois, older than 17) are under the jurisdiction of the police and, in some cases, may require that the alleged victim choose to make a report (e.g., a date-rape situation).

Tower (1992) notes that making the report can initially be uncomfortable for school professionals and suggests a number of steps, including the following, that may be useful to consider before making the call:

1. The facts should be documented and key points written down and organized.
2. The reporter is prepared to describe what causes him/her to suspect abuse/neglect in this case. Symptoms, possible indicators, and the child's disclosures have been noted.
3. The reporter is prepared to comment on what is known, and has been observed, about the child's relationship with his/her parents.
4. The reporter is ready to comment on concerns that other professionals within the school may have mentioned.
5. Contact information for CPS or the law enforcement agency is available on the alleged victim, and, if possible, the alleged perpetrator.
6. The principal has been, or will be, notified after the report (if this is the school's policy).
7. The reporter has a "debriefing" session with colleagues planned, if needed.

Going through the Principal

Thus, legal mandates require that school personnel make reports to CPS authorities and/or local police departments. In practice, however, many schools have policies or common practices in which all reports must go through the principal. Under this arrangement, teachers and other school personnel are asked to discuss suspected abuse with the principal, who will then decide whether to make the report (Zellman, 1990). One national sample of teachers found that the vast majority make their reports to the principal (Abrahams, Casey, & Daro, 1992). Similarly, a Kansas study found that none of the teachers in the sample reported directly to CPS, as mandated by law (Shoop & Firestone, 1988). Some schools have institutionalized the process of having someone else, but not necessarily the principal, make the reports. Response teams or designated receivers are appointed at some schools to review teacher suspicions and make decisions on reporting (Crenshaw, Crenshaw, & Lichtenberg, 1995).

Though common, this practice is not ideal, and in some states it may be illegal. Certainly one concern is that the procedure may delay the call. For example, what if a principal is not available at the time of the teacher's initial concern? What if the response team cannot meet for several days? Additionally, a second- or third-hand report may be less clear. The principal or other designated representative who makes the call, when questioned by the hotline worker, may not have all of the information or may be less clear than the person who actually saw the injury or heard the child's disclosure.

Perhaps the biggest concern, however, is that, by having to go through some type of gatekeeper system, some cases may not be reported that should be. For example, while response teams might seem to improve the quality of reports, they may lead educators to talk themselves out of reporting (Crenshaw et al., 1995). Principals or other administrators, when placed into a gatekeeper role, may also decide not to report. Teachers in one focus group (Crenshaw et al., 1995) placed a great deal of emphasis on administrators' tending to discourage reports; some teachers even indicated that, in their experience, administrators "overtly suppressed reports" (Crenshaw et al., 1995).

Again, such practices may not meet legal requirements on at least two levels. First, in many states it is specifically illegal for an administrator or supervisor to suppress, change, or edit a report (IDCFS, 1998). Second, "mandated reporters remain liable for their suspicions even if they have reported to their designated receiver" (Crenshaw et al., 1995, p. 1110). Thus, if a teacher suspects that a child is being maltreated and reports this to his/her principal, who thereupon disagrees and will not report it, the teacher is still mandated to report. If a report is not made, the teacher is still the one who could be charged with the failure to report, who has violated his/her professional ethics, and who may feel morally culpable. In one compelling, tragic example, Tower (1987) reports a teacher's experience:

> "I knew Henry was being beaten by his mother. My colleagues knew it too, and each one had approached the principal individually. Finally, after Henry received a particularly bad beating, I pleaded with the principal to allow me to report. When he flatly refused, I felt I had no recourse. Several days later Henry did not come to school. When I arrived home, my husband greeted me with the evening paper. Henry was dead—a victim of child abuse." (p. 52)

Just to be clear, it is quite a different matter to notify the supervisor or principal that a report has already been made (IDCFS, 1998). In fact, in most cases this is quite appropriate, because, depending on the nature of the report, CPS, police, and/or parents may soon be converging on the school, and principals should be prepared to respond accordingly.

In sum, since some states require direct reports from the person who suspects abuse, and most others prefer that CPS hear directly from the professional closest to the situation, the gatekeeper role may not meet legal requirements. This is especially true if the designee routinely fails to report situations that others believe are reportable. Since this appears to be such a common practice, state law and school district policy should be closely examined to ensure a proper level of compliance. In-service training for administrators, teachers, and other school professionals may prove helpful (Brassard et al., 1983).

Should Parents Be Informed?

While principals should not necessarily be in a gatekeeper role, it is generally appropriate to inform them of reports made by school personnel. Is this true for parents as well? Should they be informed, though not allowed to "veto" a report? This common question is a subject of considerable disagreement among professionals. State law does not require professionals to inform parents, and opinions are mixed over whether doing so would be the proper professional and ethical response.

Some argue that there are critical ethical reasons for informing the parents. If a report is made "behind their backs," this may destroy any long-term trust that the parents may have developed with the specific professional and the school more generally. Parents may be made to wonder, "*What else* is the school not telling me?" This parental attitude certainly would not be in the best interest of the child or children involved since positive home–school relationships are so important in a child's education (Christenson, 1995).

A second reason for informing parents is that they may find out anyway, so being upfront and direct is preferable. While CPS investigators do not normally inform parents of who made the report, often it is not difficult for parents to figure out who might have done so. Parents may know their child regularly sees a counselor at school, has just undergone a psychoeducational evaluation, or has been spending extra time with a particular teacher. Parents may begin to speculate that in these settings, their children may have discussed what is going on at home, or the professionals may have otherwise gained information that led them to make a report. In many cases children may tell their parents, either on their own or after parents inquire, to whom they disclosed. Thus, many argue, since parents are likely to find out anyway, they should hear it first from the school professional (IDCFS, 1998). While parents may be upset when a school professional directly informs them that a report has been made, this reaction may be mild as compared to their anger should they later learn from someone else what occurred.

But it is partially this potentially explosive emotional reaction that has led others to argue against informing parents of the report, especially in cases in which one or both parents are the suspected perpetrators. Professionals, from this point of view, fear avoidant or hostile responses from the parents. More importantly, they argue that advance notice that a report has been made may "tip off" parents to cover up the abuse, pressure the child to recant, or even physically pull up stakes and move, making an accurate investigation unlikely. Typically CPS prefers that the alleged perpetrators not be informed before its investigators can make contact.

Clearly there are convincing arguments on both sides. Decisions should be made on a case-by-base basis. Consider, for example, how different the decision might be in the following two scenarios. In one case, the school psychologist has been working with a mother in a parenting class. One day, in a private follow-up session, the mother admits that she has "lost her cool" on more than one occasion, even leaving bruises where she slapped her children's faces. The school psychologist might likely tell the mother, right then, of the need to make a report. In fact, the school psychologist might give the mother the option of making the call herself right then or staying there while the school psychologist makes the call. Quite differently, if a child reports to a teacher that she is being molested at home, that her father has movies he has made of her and her friends naked, and that her mother knows about this, the teacher will likely call the CPS hotline immediately without telling the parents. Thus, parents are not given the opportunity to hide or destroy critical evidence. A "child's safety should always be an important factor in deciding whether or not to inform the parent of your report" (IDCFS, 1998, p. 16).

What to Include in a Report?

When making the hotline call, it is generally helpful to have the required information readily available. Basic information (e.g., name, address, date of birth) regarding the child(ren) and names and contact information for the parents will be important. Additionally, specifics regarding the suspected abuse or neglect should be written down to be readily shared with the hotline worker. For example, what is the nature and extent of the injury that you observed? What did the child say about the injuries? What behaviors have you observed that may be related? Has there been a pattern of suspicious injuries and/or possibly abuse-related behaviors? Whether a child made specific disclosures or answered in a suspicious or inconsistent way when asked about injuries, it is helpful to have exact quotes of the child. If there is a specifically alleged perpetrator, the name(s) and any contact or location information may be critical. Finally, reporters should provide information about themselves and where and when investigators can contact them. In some states with overloaded hotlines, if there is not an imminently dangerous situation, the operators may need to call the reporter back several hours later. Thus, home contact information may be important to share as well. In most states, after the initial oral report is filed, a written report must follow within the next 48 hours.

When a Report Is Not Taken

As noted above, hotlines are frequently extremely busy, and workers may ask to call reporters back unless there is imminent danger. This in no way indicates that the report will not be taken, but simply that the system is overburdened. The reporter can expect a call back within a few hours.

In other instances, the child protection worker may not accept the report. Mandated reporters are often upset by this and confused as to why this would be the response. There may be a number of reasons, so it is important to seek clarification from the hotline worker.

At times, the child protection worker may not agree with the mandated reporter that this is a reportable situation. While school professionals may be thinking about "best practice" standards, CPS may be considering "minimally acceptable parenting standards." For example, the school psychologist may believe that corporal punishment is abusive as a parenting technique; however, child protection may not accept such calls unless a weapon is used, there are bruises or marks, or this is a repeated, severe pattern. Thus, some of the discrepancies may be due to different ways of thinking between, for example, mental health professionals—who may be considering ideals, clinical speculation, and intuition—and child protection workers—who must think more about evidence and legal issues (Deisz, Doueck, George, & Levine, 1996).

At other times, the reason for not taking the report is more than simply understandable differences between the professions' perspectives. At times, the hotline worker is simply incorrect. Reporting rates have skyrocketed in recent years. CPS departments are frequently overwhelmed and underfunded. It is difficult to keep up with hotline staffing demands. Individual workers, even with the best of intentions, may be inexperienced and undertrained. Thus, if school professionals disagree with the worker's decision, they should feel free to ask for a supervisor.

Even if there is a decision not to take the report, CPS will typically keep records of the call on file for 6 months. Thus, if the professional gains additional information that may "tip the scale," this could be added to the original report (IDCFS, 1998). Others may also make independent reports that, when compiled collectively, yield enough information for an investigation.

FAILURE TO REPORT

School personnel, as a professional group, are responsible for the largest number of reports (DHHS, 1999). On the surface, this may appear to indicate that educators are clearly following the mandate to report all suspected abuse and neglect. However, compared to most other sources, school personnel have much more contact and thus more information about many children, so initial conclusions about reporting compliance may be misleading. In fact, there is reason to believe that schools are also responsible for the largest number of *failures* to report (O'Toole et al., 1999; Crenshaw et al., 1995).

The available information regarding reporting and nonreporting rates and rationales is based primarily on three types of studies. Some questionnaires directly ask general mandated reporters or educators specifically to describe their reporting patterns and decisions. In other methodologies, respondents are asked to consider case vignettes and make hypothetical reporting decisions. Finally, focus group discussions have allowed investigators to develop a more qualitative understanding of the reporting decision process. These sources of information, combined with government reporting statistics, have provided some important information for consideration.

For example, in one questionnaire study, a sizable number of elementary and middle school teachers (36–53%, depending on type of maltreatment asked about) indicated that they had not suspected any cases of child abuse during the preceding two school years (Crenshaw et al., 1995). Even larger numbers (50–76%) made no reports. The authors of the study, extrapolating the number of students, on average, that teachers instruct per year with abuse rates, point out that most teachers would teach between 6 (elementary) and 30 (middle school) abused children over a 2-year period. They raise the question of how teachers could not have suspected and/or reported any abuse during that time (Crenshaw et al., 1995).

In another study of mandated reporters, 40% of respondents clearly acknowledged that, at some time in their career, they had suspected abuse or neglect but had decided not to report it (Zellman & Faller, 1996). A study specific to school psychologists found that only 61% of respondents presented with a reportable case vignette indicated they would report it (Wilson & Gettinger, 1989).

Those Who Do Report

In order to understand why some mandated reporters do not report, it may be helpful to consider the rationales of those who do report. Those who report abuse indicate that they do so for a variety of reasons, citing specifically the hope that the report will help stop the maltreatment (Zellman & Faller, 1996). Those most likely to report have the attitude that the school is the "first line of defense against abuse and neglect" (Crenshaw et al., 1995, p. 1106). Reporters also cite the fact that the law requires reporting (Zellman & Faller, 1996). In general, educators do know the law and typically desire to adhere to it (Crenshaw et al., 1995).

Decisions about reporting may also be related to specifics about the suspected abuse. Reports are more likely to be made if the abuse is thought to be severe and occurring presently, the victim is young and female, and there is a history of maltreatment. Suspected physical abuse, compared to other forms of child maltreatment, is most likely to be reported, followed by sexual abuse, neglect, and emotional abuse (Crenshaw et al., 1995; Wilson & Gettinger, 1989; Zellman & Faller, 1996). In one study, for example, 78% of suspected physical abuse was reported, followed by 66% of sexual abuse, 40% of neglect, and 22% of emotional abuse (Crenshaw et al., 1995).

Those Who Do Not Report

While mandated to report, many professionals are reluctant to do so for a variety of reasons (Johnson, 1989). Rationales for failure to report can be grouped into five categories: fears, lack of information/expertise, school-related obstacles, problems with CPS, and concerns about the child. Following is a brief discussion and a "rebuttal" to each excuse.

Fears

Frequently, it is the mandated reporters' fears that keep them from reporting. In many cases, school professionals are most afraid of the potentially angry or hostile response of parents (Tower, 1992). Thus, school mental health professionals or teachers may be reluctant to get involved, fearing parents will take retribution physically or legally (Reiniger, Robison, & McHugh, 1995). They may fear they will be legally liable if the investigation does not confirm abuse. Even if they do not anticipate an overtly hostile reaction from a particular family in question, school professionals may feel awkward. They may fear that the report will cause extreme discomfort, particularly if they know the family well and/or the parents are respected in the school community (Tower, 1992; Zellman & Faller, 1996).

Another fear is related to getting involved with the whole child protection system. For some, it is primarily a fear of testifying in court. For others, it is a more pragmatic fear, as they are concerned about the "hassle" and time commitment involved in engaging the child protection system (Reiniger et al., 1995; Zellman & Faller, 1996).

Fears may in some cases lead to school personnel intentionally suppressing a report. "I really do think this child is being abused by his father, but that man is scary, and there is no way I am calling in a report and risking my own life." Other times, fears may have a more subtle influence, as school professionals simply do not allow themselves to detect or suspect abuse. They may do this by not looking closely enough, not asking questions, or taking the "I see nothing" approach (IDCFS, 1998).

Response to Fears

Such fears are understandable. However, for the sake of children's well-being, school professionals must move beyond them. The following information may be helpful.

Concerns about legal retribution should be allayed by the reminder that "State law protects the identity of all mandated reporters, and you are given immunity from legal liability as a result of reports you make in good faith" (IDCFS, 1998, p. 5).

Concerns regarding physical danger are also understandable, given that part of what may be the concern is the violence of a parent. The National Center on Child Abuse and Neglect report for educators addresses this concern:

> Teachers often ask if they are in personal danger. Although there may be very few exceptions, most abusive parents lack the social skills to face adults, especially those whom they perceive to be in authority positions. This feeling of not being able to confront adults is exactly the reason why abusive parents turn their anger or frustration toward the child(ren) or their spouse. An occasional parent may yell or threaten but that is usually as far as it goes. Thus, educators should be assured that in most cases they are in no danger. (Tower, 1992, p. 38)

Additionally, if adult educators are fearful of a parent, one can imagine how the dependent children of this person must feel. This fear, while uncomfortable, may help the school professional empathize with the child and be even more motivated to report. "If I, as a 40-year-old professional, independent adult am terrified of this man, what must his 5-year-old son be feeling?"

Similarly, the less serious concerns regarding the time, hassle, or awkwardness must be put into the same perspective. Individuals must ask themselves, "Compared to what the child may be enduring, is a small investment of my time, although inconvenient, really too much to give?"

Lack of Information/Expertise

A second obstacle to reporting is school professionals' lack of information or confidence in their decisions. While most mandated reporters, including educators, are familiar with the basics of the reporting law, there remains some apparent confusion that keeps them from reporting (IDCFS, 1998).

Educators openly admit their lack of information and confidence. Crenshaw and colleagues (1995) found that only 10% of educators felt very well prepared to recognize and report child abuse, while only another 51% felt fairly well prepared. The remaining 40% felt barely adequate, poorly, or not at all prepared. Teachers were especially likely to fall into the lower categories.

Much of the confusion relates to the language. Potential reporters are confused by vague phrases such as "reasonable cause," "excessive corporal punishment," and "substantial risk of harm" that appear in reporting laws (Deisz et al., 1996). For example, many school professionals may not endorse any form of corporal punishment but recognize that this would not be considered reportable abuse. Yet, at what point does it become such? When bruises or marks are left? When a "weapon" is used? Terms such as "reasonable cause to believe" or "reason to suspect" are also subject to some interpretation. Should every "hunch" be reported? How much evidence is required? While most would agree that not every intuitive guess is reportable, too many mandated reporters do not report when they should because they believe the situation is not serious enough (Zellman & Faller, 1996) or they are waiting for more conclusive evidence.

Additionally, in an effort to be sensitive to diversity, others question their rights to intervene by reporting, especially when there are potentially cultural differences. For example, one teacher in the NCCAN Report for Educators (Tower, 1992) questioned her role: " 'In their country hitting the children severely is accepted practice,' she said, 'What right do I have to tell them to change their cultural values?' " (p. 38).

Response to Lack of Information/Expertise

A lack of confidence in understanding the details of the reporting law, the exact interpretation of the legal language, or the best response to families of diverse backgrounds who may be abusing their children may be understandable. However, it is important that these uncertainties not be used to avoid or unnecessarily delay reports that should be made.

In-service training should be provided to teachers to present additional information and answer questions regarding reporting obligations. Most educators understand that, by law, they are mandated reporters; yet, there may be need for additional information regarding the threshold of "reason to suspect" as well as practical advice on interpreting other somewhat ambiguous aspects of the law. Additionally, training might address how schools can combine the goal of respecting differences in cultures with protecting the safety of children.

At times, the "excuse" of "lack of information" may be more related to the first reason for not reporting, that is, fear. Educators should be encouraged to engage in some self-examination. "Is it really that I do not understand my obligation to report in this situation, or am I afraid?" If it is honestly as simple as "I really do not know if this situation is reportable," a call can always be made, the situation described, and CPS can help the educator determine whether the threshold has been crossed.

School-Related Obstacles

Related to the concern regarding lack of information, a paucity of child abuse report training provided to educators is one frequently cited concern (Tower, 1992). Too many educators receive little, if any, training in college, and then perhaps only a brief lecture in their new-teacher orientation program.

An additional school-related obstacle, as discussed earlier, is the tendency of some administrators to interfere with reporting. Again, this may be illegal and certainly puts teachers and other school personnel in a bind (Tower, 1992).

Response to School-Related Obstacles

Schools should make ongoing training, supervision, and support for child abuse reporting available. Administrators as well as teachers should be included in the training so that "gatekeeper" arrangements that interfere with reporting are discontinued and that teachers feel supported, not discouraged, by their supervisors when making child abuse reports. Given the fears and questions that already exist, educators do not need the extra burden of feeling that they will have to go through, or against, their employer's preferences to do what they feel legally, ethically, or morally obligated to do.

Problems with CPS

Perhaps even more frequently disturbing than the obstacles one encounters within the schools are mandated reporters' distrust of CPS. Many simply do not trust the protective agency to respond appropriately. Mandated reporters report past negative experiences with CPS as reasons for their later reluctance to report (IDCFS, 1998). The concerns expressed include that previous reports did no good or resulted in overreactions or underreactions (Tower, 1992; Zellman & Faller, 1996).

Response to Problems with CPS

The *NCCAN User Manual for Educators* acknowledges that such concerns are real and valid but points out that "a previous bad experience does not mean that the next time the case will not be handled well" since in many states CPS agencies are becoming more skilled and responsive (Tower, 1992, p. 39). Additionally, school professionals must keep the larger picture in mind. It is only through public disclosure of child maltreatment and the involvement of social agencies that the abusive cycle may be broken and the healing cycle may begin (Johnson, 1989). Accurate reporting rates will potentially increase funding and enhance policy decisions so that future cases will be more appropriately addressed. Educators who report truly legitimate concerns at least have fulfilled their obligation. They have done what they can do, and then, hopefully, CPS will perform its role adequately.

Child-Related Concerns

This concern about CPS, however, is very closely tied to the last and perhaps most difficult issue: concern about the child. If CPS mishandles the case, educators may fear there will be no enforcement, just enough agency involvement to get the child in further trouble, or an overreaction by the system that will end in having the child pulled from secure, positive experiences such as school due to an out-of-home placement (Johnson, 1989). In sum, there is a fear that reporting will retraumatize the child.

Additionally, for mental health providers, there are concerns that a report would disrupt treatment. Breaking confidentiality is a serious decision. According to state laws, "Privileged communication between professional and client is not grounds for failure to report" (IDCFS, 1998, p. 5). However, this does not make the decision easy for a school psychologist who is working with an adolescent who has begged the psychologist not to tell (especially if the abuse was mild and unlikely to receive significant attention from an overburdened CPS), or a parent who has admitted physical abuse but is clearly working on the problem (and would likely leave treatment, and therefore not be monitored, if a report were made).

Response to Child-Related Concerns

When a professional genuinely believes that it is in the best interest of a child to not make the report, the dilemma is most serious and legitimate. While these dilemmas are certainly difficult, educators must be clear that to not report well-founded suspicions is to break the law. At this point reporting laws do not allow for discretionary reporting (in which mental health providers would be allowed some latitude), although some observers (Zellman & Faller, 1996) have called for it.

Perhaps a solution is for school administrators to develop a closer working relationship with CPS so that, rather than going through the hotline, school professionals can speak with the local CPS office regarding a particularly sensitive case. Additionally, educators are urged to ask an agency supervisor to intervene if there are ongoing concerns about a particular case (Tower, 1992). "While reporting does not guarantee that the situation will improve, *not* reporting guarantees that the child will continue to be at risk if abuse or neglect exists" (Tower, 1992, p. 39).

While there may be some risks in reporting, there are also many risks, both legal and ethical, for not reporting suspected abuse. Imagine, for example, a case in which a school psychologist does not report the suspected physical abuse of a child due to some of the fears discussed above, and later the child is more severely injured, or even killed.

Solutions

Clearly, there is a high incidence of failures to report, and many rationales that have led to these decisions. While certain arguments in rebuttal were discussed earlier, here are some additional specific suggestions:

1. The CPS hotline can be used for informational purposes. If educators are not clear about whether their concern crosses a reasonable threshold of suspicion, they may, without giving their name or the name of the children they are concerned about, call in hypothetical situations (Deisz et al., 1996).

2. Training must be provided on an ongoing basis. Future training must go beyond merely reciting the basic reporting law and providing the hotline numbers. Too often educators are aware of the law, yet are still inconsistent in their reporting. Thus, "there is no evidence for the oft-cited conclusion that improving the knowledge, understanding, and support of mandatory reporting will increase reporting tendency and rate" (Crenshaw et al., 1995, p. 1111). Training must teach educators "to look at themselves as a first line of defense against child abuse, how to achieve reasonable suspicion, and ways to avoid extraneous issues which should not impact on their decision" (Crenshaw et al., 1995, p. 1111).

School professionals should be trained specifically on how best to collaborate with CPS. In fact, CPS representatives should be frequently invited to the school to provide training to teachers and to answer their questions.

3. Ongoing support from and consultation with peers and supervisors should be encouraged. Clearly, there are numerous emotional issues (e.g., fears, frustrations) that interfere with good reporting decisions. School professionals should create systems in which there are opportunities to be supported and should move beyond emotional reactions in order to make good decisions. Thus, peers and supervisors should be consulted in helping determine whether an abuse report should be made. It should be noted, however, that if a professional is consulting with a colleague about whether or not he/she should report an incident or situation, it is quite likely that there is already some reason to suspect abuse or neglect.

4. Developing more collaborative relationships with CPS departments and individual workers is critical. In one focus group study, when CPS knew and trusted the mandated reporter making the call, they considered the reports more seriously (Deisz et al., 1996). Some school professionals may be creating obstacles in the relationships by talking to the CPS workers in an ad-

versarial or condescending way (due to pedantic attitudes, perhaps, regard-ing education, professional experience, etc.) or using clinical jargon (Deisz et al., 1996). A positive alternative is setting up formal and informal meetings to discuss concerns and develop effective working relationships (Deisz et al., 1996). "What is more important at this time is for school psychologists (and other school personnel) to develop cooperative, working relationships with the county agency and to view agency workers as individuals who are also striving to provide the best services to abused children" (Wilson & Gettinger, 1989, p. 100).

AFTER THE REPORT

Addressing the Child

After a report has been made, it is again important for the school profession-al to explain to the child, as much as possible, what can be anticipated. The school professional will still not be able to say exactly how a child protection agency will proceed, but experience and an ongoing relationship with these agencies will help the professional to have some idea of the likely response for various types of abuse reports. For example, a school psychologist who has made a report after a young child disclosed sexual abuse by a neighbor might explain, "I told the police, and I told your mom, about what you told me. Everyone is very concerned. The police said they may come to school or to your house to talk to you, or you might go with your mom to a special place called a Child's Advocacy Center to talk to them. The police wanting to talk to you does not mean you are in trouble. They will be trying to find out what happened and help you."

Recall another aspect of informing the child about what he/she can an-ticipate next is to be clear with the child about what he/she can expect from school professionals. Once again, school mental health professionals are urged to be sensitive and compassionate, yet realistic about what can be of-fered, given the many children (with a variety of needs) who they serve. Mak-ing and keeping reasonable commitments to a child is actually more caring than making grandiose promises that will have to be broken.

Hearing Outcomes

School professionals who make reports of abuse are often frustrated that they do not hear of any outcomes. They have often been left asking, "What hap-pened? Don't they ever do anything? Didn't they believe the child? Was my time wasted?" Certainly, confidentiality concerns keep CPS from sharing de-tails of investigations with school professionals; however, many states are now allowing educators and other mandated reporters to at least learn of the outcome of specific investigations. This notification typically comes in the form of a letter that documents whether the report was "indicated" or "unfounded." "Indicated" or in some states "substantiated" cases are those for which CPS could find credible evidence to support the allegation of abuse or neglect.

Since many reports are "unfounded" or "not substantiated," it is important that school professionals understand that a report's not being substantiated does not necessarily mean that abuse did not occur or that a report was inappropriate. Reports may be unfounded or not substantiated for numerous reasons, including a lack of information (e.g., the child is vague about who was abusive, and no one else can corroborate) and situations in which the child is no longer at risk (e.g., an abusive boyfriend has moved out of state) (Zellman & Faller, 1996). At times, however, the report is not substantiated due to CPS's errors. For that reason, in most states school personnel can appeal an investigation outcome and ask that the case be reconsidered. Additionally, school personnel are reminded that, as more information is gained in situations previously resulting in "unfounded" outcomes (e.g., additional child disclosures, more injuries), new reports should be made. In some cases it is only after a series of reports with enough additional specifics have been made that CPS has enough information to adequately investigate, substantiate, and take action to protect children.

CONCLUSION

Reporting is the not the end of the response to child abuse and neglect. In fact, "concentrating societal effort on reporting, while at the same time neglecting intervention, makes little sense and is cruel to children and families affected" (O'Toole et al., 1999, p. 1098). Reporting, however, can be the means to intervention. While school professionals are to be congratulated for being frequent reporters of abuse, there should be serious concern about the degree of underreporting by school personnel. It is critical that educators recognize the unique opportunity they have to detect evidence of maltreatment and report well-grounded suspicions. Legal, ethical, and moral rationales are clear. Such obstacles as fear, confusion, or systemic problems must be addressed so that children can be better protected against abuse or neglect.

CHAPTER 4

♦♦♦

Treatment Referrals

♦

with AMY GENRICH

SHOULD DIRECT INTERVENTION BE PROVIDED BY THE SCHOOLS?

Over the years there have been debates in various professional literatures regarding the appropriateness of providing family therapy, or counseling in general, in the schools. Some have believed that these mental health services are beyond the role of school professionals and not suited for the academic context. Others have argued that, if there are clear education-related concerns, it may be appropriate to offer services at school. Still others have pointed out that mental health and education are inextricably intertwined. Mental health, this last perspective argues, "should not be viewed as a separate agenda from the instructional mission" (Adelman & Taylor, 1998b, p. 150).

This debate continues today. Many schools have begun attempting to improve accessibility to health and mental services by developing more school-linked and school-based services (Davis, 1997). This "Full Service School Movement" is growing, and some schools offer medical, dental, and a range of mental health services (Skinner, 1999). Proponents of these reforms (sometimes known by a variety of other related terms such as school-linked, integrated services, school-based, one-stop shopping, wraparound services, seamless service delivery, comprehensive school health, etc.; Adelman & Taylor, 1998a) point out that services should be offered where students are: at school (Dryfoos, 1994). They argue that "mental health and psychosocial problems must be addressed if schools are to function satisfactorily and if students are to learn effectively" (Adelman & Taylor, 1998b, p. 150).

Amy Genrich is a doctoral candidate in the School Psychology Program at Illinois State University, Normal, Illinois.

Those opposed are calling for a "back to basics" approach in which schools narrow their focus to academic concerns. Opposition to expanding into other areas (e.g., mental health concerns) is based on two primary issues. First, there is concern that schools are losing their primary mission: academics. Time, money, and staff resources spent on counseling, for example, are not spent on teaching. Second, some have raised concerns that schools expanding into the medical and mental health arenas may be infringing on family rights and values. These concerns are especially heightened if schools are involved in sex education and sexuality curricula (Adelman & Taylor, 1998b; Davis, 1997).

In addition to the broader questions regarding schools providing mental health services, various professional groups are having their own "role and function" discussions. School psychologists, for example, while traditionally having duties focused primarily on assessment roles, are moving to more mental health related functions. Most are prepared to do some counseling; many enjoy the role (Fagan & Wise, 1994). There is support by many to continue to develop a more expanded role, as evidenced by the following position statement:

> Although there are clear limits in the skills any professional can master and deliver, given the breadth and depth of current problems facing our children, school psychologists' role and function should never be reduced to either-or decision making. Rather, if we are to address seriously mental health problems facing our children, information, procedures, and theory directed at prevention and remediation of school-based problems should not be excluded from school psychologists' role and function. . . . Schools need some mental health professionals with expertise and training across a wide variety of interventions and prevention procedures. (Skinner, 1999, p. 193)

With such a range of responses to the more general questions about school-based mental health services, and the roles of school psychologists, it may not be surprising that there could be a range of answers to the question "Is it appropriate for schools to provide counseling or therapy services for children have been victims of child maltreatment?" While some might have a quick answer based on their position on the issues above, a more thoughtful response, however, must be made on a case-by-case basis, first considering the answers to a number of other questions.

Questions to Consider

There are several possible treatment options: the child may receive primary services outside of the school, at the school, or some combination of both.

When choosing which option would be most appropriate, the school-based practitioner or multidisciplinary team should consider several issues. The specific needs of the child should be kept in mind when deciding treatment, based on the following influences: community factors (e.g., other available options), institutional factors (e.g., administration, support, district philosophy), school practitioner factors (e.g., expertise, available time), family factors (e.g., family, residence of the child, denial/acceptance) and student factors (e.g., the student's own assessment of severity). Table 4.1 provides a list of guiding questions to be answered for each of these factors when determining the appropriateness of school-based treatment. It is important to remember that treatment decisions should be made on a case-by-case basis.

TABLE 4.1. Questions to Consider When Deciding Whether to Provide Therapeutic Services at School

Community resource factors

- What services are available in the community?
- Is the student already receiving services from a community provider?
- Does that community provider want school involvement?

Institutional factors

- Do the school's administrators philosophically support providing more intensive therapy to students in school?
- Do teachers agree that students should occasionally miss class for such purposes?
- Is there space for such activities to occur?
- Is there school legal support to consult?

School practitioner factors

- Does the school mental health practitioner want to be involved in this type of work?
- Has the person who will be providing the services had sufficient training in therapeutic interventions, particularly with child maltreatment issues?
- Is there supervision available to the person who will be providing the services in school?
- Is the school practitioner's workload and current level of stress at a point at which working with traumatized clients would not be "too much"?

Family factors

- Does the child's family support the provision of services in the school?
- Is the child's family confronting the abuse or neglect, or are family members in denial?
- Is the child still residing in a dangerous situation?
- Does the child interact with the former perpetrator?
- If services are not provided in the school, will the family seek outside services?

Student factors

- Does the student want services?
- Does the student want services in the school setting? How are his/her studies going?
- How severe are the student's problems?
- Is the student a danger to self or others?

Community Factors

Perhaps one of the first factors to consider is essentially "What is the alternative?" It is important to consider what other options are available in the community. Additionally, before rushing to supply school-based services, it is advisable to find out if the child or the family is already receiving community-based services. If they are, it is important to consider whether the outside clinician is open to the possibility of school-based mental health services as an additional support or whether the other professional would view the additional services as redundant, or even in conflict.

Institutional Factors

The most obvious institutional factor is the administration. The support or lack of support for providing mental health services in general—and addressing child maltreatment issues in particular—is a critical consideration. Whether it is child abuse prevention programs or individual therapy with victims, child maltreatment is a controversial issue to many administrators. Administrators may fear that addressing the subject at any level can lead to allegations, upset parents, and lawsuits, which are precisely the situations they most strive to avoid. A clear understanding of the administration's philosophy and mission statement would be helpful for the team to know. A district that has just adopted a "back to the basics" approach will have a very different view of serving maltreated children than one that is interested in broadening the role of schools in children's lives.

A less obvious but still very important influence on treatment success is the support of teachers. Teachers hold the key to accessing the students. Accountability standards for teachers are rising, which means teachers are being expected to instruct children effectively on a vast amount of material within a given time frame. Because of this expectation, and perhaps the potential disruption that may result in their classrooms, teachers are not always eager to have students pulled from instruction in order to receive special services. For this reason, teacher support is critical to maintaining consistent contact with a child in the school setting. In-service training for teachers and administrators on child maltreatment issues and the proposed intervention plan should be considered. Professionals who are well informed about the prevalence and effects of child abuse are likely to be most supportive of counseling services being provided at school.

School Practitioner Factors

Not all school practitioners will be interested in providing abuse-focused services, as these require some degree of specialization (Vevier & Tharinger,

1986). Thus, the first consideration for the school-based clinician is "Do you want to do this?" The desire to be involved in these issues is an important consideration. Second, the school-based practitioner should consider whether he/she has adequate training to perform in such a role. Questions regarding prior professional experience, university coursework and practicum, and continuing education experiences should be considered. If it is a stretch to one's professional competence, is adequate supervision available?

Additionally, working with children who have been maltreated can be very emotionally intense. School practitioners who are already professionally overloaded and/or experiencing significant personal stressors may be wise to refer a highly traumatized student to another clinician.

Family Factors

Family circumstances constitute the key environmental factors for most children. The family's support of school services, who the child lives with, the amount of contact the child has with the perpetrator, and the family's likelihood of obtaining outside services for the child should all be assessed prior to committing to providing services in the school. Practical concerns such as the family's financial resources, including insurance, as well as transportation access, should also be considered.

Student Factors

The nature and severity of the student's reasons for referral should, of course, be a consideration in deciding where the child should be served. A child with intense psychological needs might be best served off campus, if possible, and in some cases he/she may be placed in a therapeutic school and/or residential placement. Certainly if the child is a danger to him/herself or others, precautions must be taken to protect all involved. School services may still be most appropriate for this child, but safety must be a high priority for all involved.

The student's view of receiving services in the school can be a fundamental component of planning for success. If the child is embarrassed to have therapy in school for fear that friends or teachers will learn the details of his/her life, services should not be conducted in the school or great care should be taken to ensure privacy. Beyond finding a private space to meet and treating the sessions confidentially, school-based mental health professionals should consider a reasonable way to excuse the child from class (without revealing the nature of the excuse). Additionally, whether missing class is a wise idea should be evaluated. How is the student doing academically? Would missed class time be a problem?

Hypothetical cases may be used to illustrate how best practices may vary on a case-by-case basis. Consider, for example, a 9-year-old boy, Jason, who, after being asked about some recent sexual behavior at school, disclosed to the school psychologist that he had been sexually abused by a babysitter. The school psychologist reported this disclosure to both the CPS and to Jason's parents. The parents, though certainly upset, responded absolutely appropriately. They believed Jason, took action to ensure no further contact with the babysitter, and promptly followed up on the school psychologist's referral to a local psychologist who specializes in treating sexual abuse victims, including sexual behavior problems. Initial word back from that psychologist was that, from her point of view, Jason's treatment was going well, but she would welcome any feedback from the school. Teacher reports indicated that the sexual gestures had stopped completely and that Jason was succeeding in the third grade.

Quite differently, imagine a young adolescent female, Maria, who was severely sexually abused by her stepfather. She disclosed her experience to a teacher after a prevention program. Although the case was founded by CPS and the father was convicted and imprisoned, Maria's mother does not support her daughter. She says that, if this really did happen, it was Maria's fault. She is angry with Maria for reporting and "causing all of these problems." Without her husband's income, Ms. Ramirez is forced to work two jobs to support the four children. Maria's mother is careful to say enough of the "right" things to avoid any future CPS involvement, but she is certainly not likely to follow up on any counseling referrals for herself or for Maria that have been repeatedly made by both CPS and the school psychologist. Maria is a bright teen who is doing amazingly well, given all that she has endured; she has a 3.0 GPA and is one semester away from graduation. One day Maria surprises a teacher by confiding that she has thought about dropping out of school. Maria says she feels guilty. She wonders if maybe her mother is right—maybe she did cause the abuse, maybe the least she could do is work full time to help support the family.

Notice how different the decisions might be regarding the appropriateness of the school providing therapeutic services. Jason seems to be getting all that he needs from an outside source. Beyond providing the psychologist with school-based feedback, there may be no need for school involvement. Quite differently, Maria is not getting what she needs and does not appear to be likely to get mental health services from any outside source. More referrals for outside services are likely to be met with the same passive resistance. The emotional and cognitive effects of the abuse and the aftermath are having a serious impact on Maria's academic decision making. In a case like this, school-based intervention seems clearly the reasonable, compassionate response.

Once it is determined that the school may have a role in providing mental health interventions for children and adolescents who have been maltreated, there are a variety of options to consider. Many students with a history of abuse may benefit from other, general mental health counseling. Some might be included in groups specifically for children who have been abused. Finally, individual abuse-focused counseling may be provided to some children.

Although there are numerous factors to consider when deciding the best treatment for the child, the aforementioned obstacles are not intended to be overwhelming or to dissuade school staff from providing services to abused and/or neglected children. The information is provided as a "heads up" so that any interventions for the student can be as successful as possible.

MAKING A REFERRAL TO AN OUTSIDE AGENCY

The following discussion regarding making outside treatment referrals is not exclusively for schools who do not provide therapeutic services to children and adolescents. Even full-service or therapeutic schools must on occasion refer students to other clinicians.

Consider the following scenario. Jody and Jenny report to their mother that they have been sexually abused by their babysitter, a family friend, for the past 2 years. Soon after the disclosure, their mother, Ms. Rose, calls each of the girls' schools to let someone know what has occurred and to seek advice. At both schools her call is forwarded to the school psychologist. Ms. Rose feels guilty about having left her children with this person and not having known that someone was hurting them. Ms. Rose was also molested when she was a child, so her daughters' recent disclosure has brought up a lot of memories and feelings for her, causing her additional distress. On the phone, Ms. Rose sounds like she is feeling overwhelmed by all that has happened.

For various reasons, both school psychologists decide to refer Ms. Rose to an outside mental health provider for services. Jenny's school psychologist, Mr. McMillan, flips through the phone book while on the telephone with Ms. Rose, and gives her the names of two therapists who work with children. Jody's school psychologist, Mr. Stevenson, asks Ms. Rose to come to school for a meeting, during which they discuss how the girls are doing, how Ms. Rose is coping, support for the family, what services Ms. Rose would like for her children, and what each member of the family needs. Together Ms. Rose and Mr. Stevenson choose the outside services they prefer after discussing the characteristics and advantages and disadvantages of each. Although Ms. Rose appeared to be in a better position to process what is happening than when she first called, it was apparent to Mr. Stevenson that she was still overwhelmed by the recent disclosure, what it had brought up from her own abuse history, and everyday struggles.

Having recently updated the referral files with his secretary, Mr.

Stevenson knew it could be daunting to contact the various mental health agencies, especially for someone new to the process of obtaining mental health services. As invested as Ms. Rose was in her children's lives, she still needed extra support in making the phone call. Mr. Stevenson offered Ms. Rose the opportunity to make the phone call in his office. He also gave her information for adult survivors of sexual abuse, knowing that her history could play a large part in her daughters' recovery. Finally, Mr. Stevenson offered to check in with Ms. Rose in a week and with Jody the next day. Although the two psychologists both referred the students to outside services—possibly even to the same provider—the outcomes for this family could have been very different, given the variable support and information the family received in the process.

Once a decision is made about whether to refer the child to a therapist in the community, there are numerous factors to consider that will lead to a more successful referral. Just as when trying to decide whether the child should receive services primarily at school, many issues can influence the success of the referral (e.g., if the family follows through, if the therapist is a proper match for the client). The Center for Mental Health in Schools (1997) reports that follow-through rates for referrals made by school staff are less than 50%; that is, for every 10 students that are identified as needing services and for whom an outside referral is deemed best, only 5 or fewer students are actually getting the services. Conti (1975) also found that follow-through rates were lowest for referrals made by the school to outside counseling services than for any other type of school referral. Since most of the referrals for maltreated children will involve counseling, the referrals for maltreated children are particularly susceptible to poor follow-through. This means that there are numerous students and families with unmet needs, which places them at risk for further mental health and school problems (Downing, 1985). With large numbers of students not obtaining needed services, the functioning of the school may also be disrupted. A child with unmet needs of any kind tends to take away from constructive class time, often exhibiting either disruptive behavior or lack of motivation. This indicates that anything the school can do to facilitate a successful referral will improve not only the life of an individual child but also likely the classroom of that student as well. Thus, the outcome of one student referral can affect an entire classroom of students either positively or negatively, depending on the success of the referral.

Referral practices, which are often overlooked and haphazard, can have an important impact on students. Cheston (1991) explains that the referral process is rarely discussed and is not taught in professional training, mostly because clinicians typically focus on helping clients rather than on how to pass them along to someone else. She has observed that taking the time to make an appropriate and supported referral often leads to a better match between client and clinician and better outcomes for the client (Cheston, 1991).

When choosing a referral source, characteristics of the available service providers, the family, and the child should be considered. Table 4.2 provides some questions to consider when making outside referrals.

Service Providers

Once school-based practitioners or the intervention team has decided that an outside referral is appropriate, they will need to be aware of available community resources. The characteristics of various community mental health agencies should be investigated. This can be done through a variety of methods: discussing resources with colleagues, contacting local community organizations (e.g., CHADD [Children and Adults with Attention Deficit Disorder], Parents Anonymous), contacting state mental health professional organizations (i.e., state associations for school psychologists or school counselors), or reviewing the phone book for available services. Often county

TABLE 4.2. Questions to Consider When Making an Outside Referral

Service providers

- Is there a waiting list for clients? If yes, approximately, how long is the waiting period?
- What is the cost of services?
- Is there a sliding fee scale?
- Does the agency accept insurance payments?
- What is the background of the service providers (areas of expertise, degree level)?
- What kinds of services are provided (child vs. adult, individual, group, family)?
- Does the agency employ clinicians from multiple ethnic groups?
- Are there any bilingual clinicians available?
- Does the agency have both male and female clinicians?
- How does the agency match clients to clinicians?

Family

- Is the family interested in pursuing services?
- Do they have transportation?
- What is their financial and insurance situation?
- What is the family's perception or attitude toward seeking mental health services?
- Are there any other needs, such as child care, that may affect the family's ability to follow through with services?
- Are there languages besides English spoken in the home?

Child

- What is the child's perception of mental health services?
- What is the nature of the child's problems?
- Is the child in danger from others?
- Is the child a danger to self or others?
- What is the race/ethnicity/culture of the child?
- What is the gender of the child?

mental health departments have resource lists already compiled. These lists could be used as a starting point so that school staff would only have to add to and update these existing lists. The Internet can also be a useful source. Local resources may have websites that provide details about their organization, and other websites containing general information about the effects of child maltreatment can be found. School staff can recommend particular websites to parents as another information resource. For example, the American Psychological Association (APA) has a site, *http://helping.apa.org/ forms/brochures.cfm,* which answers parents' questions about obtaining mental health services. The site also provides a phone number (800-964-2000) that school staff can use or provide to parents for finding a psychologist in any community. Importantly, school practitioners should evaluate all Internet sites themselves before suggesting them to parents or other staff.

Beyond these resource-finding techniques, firsthand knowledge of community professionals can be gained by forming working relationships with service providers. Although the time of school staff and other mental health providers is often in demand, the relationships and respect gained from serving on relevant community task forces and meeting with other community professionals will prove to be invaluable. It is these relationships that can provide the knowledge of what services are available and perhaps speedier access for clients who are referred. By participating in local task forces, professional organizations, or peer supervision groups, school professionals can develop and maintain better connections with possible referral candidates.

It is not recommended that practitioners use only one technique in gathering information on the various resources. Using only the phone book will not provide a true understanding of the approach of each agency. On the other hand, limiting referrals to agencies with which personal relationships have been formed could possibly eliminate some appropriate selections. Most likely, to develop a comprehensive list, a combination of these methods will be needed. A list of community resources should be updated periodically. Entries may be kept in a binder so that revisions can be easily made. The areas of specialization, treatment format (i.e., individual, group, or family), and treatment approach of each agency are important to include under the description of each provider. The Center for Mental Health in Schools (1997) suggests categorizing services by location of services and type of problem, such as drug/alcohol dependency or domestic violence. Also, demographic information for each organization should be listed, along with the phone number, address, cost of services, sliding-fee availability, and length of waiting list. The sample provided in Figure 4.1 illustrates one way to organize information. Formats could vary widely, based on the type of community and the various services provided.

Specific inquiries to the agency should be made just prior to providing the family with the name of a resource in order to find out the most recent

COMMUNITY RESOURCES

General Mental Health Services

Agency: **River City Mental Health**

Address: 123 River Drive

               River City

Phone :   (888) 555-0000

Fees: $80/hour

Sliding fee scale available: Yes

Description of services: Individual and family counseling is provided for various
                              mental health issues.

Other info: RCMH provides child care services by the hour while
                             families are in therapy.

Runaway Services

Agency: **A Teen's Place**

Address: Kept confidential; if you are a teen in need of help, call and A Teen's Place
               will inform you of the location.

Phone: (888) 555-1212

Fees: Free

Sliding fee scale available: NA

Description of services: A Teen's Place provides shelter/meals and counseling
                              services to teen runaways (13- to 17-year-olds).

Other info: A Teen's Place will also pick up a teen runaway from any
                             place locally.

FIGURE 4.1. Sample resource sheet.

status of services, particularly current fees, and the current length of a waiting list. At larger community mental health agencies, additional information
about the clinicians currently on staff (e.g., qualifications, race/ethnicity,
gender, bilingual abilities) should also be updated periodically.

If possible, referrals for children with sexual behavior problems should
only be made to providers with immediate openings (Horton, 1996). This im-
mediacy would be especially important for children who are sexually acting
out, but also for other maltreated children, making the length of a provider's
waiting list a high priority when considering referrals. Horton (1996) also
suggests referring to providers with expertise in a specific type of child maltreatment. Training and expertise and the relative availability of potential
providers are two issues that the school-based practitioner should emphasize

when helping families select a mental health agency. Other provider characteristics can be evaluated, based on the family's values and desires, but the importance of these two criteria should not be overlooked.

Although having referral sources available for the multidisciplinary team and school staff is important, this information should also be made accessible to those students who do not wish to confide directly with school staff. This could be accomplished by having a resource area where students could obtain names of community agencies and programs, hotline numbers, and information on various mental health issues. Additionally, laminated wallet-sized cards of key community resources and phone numbers are another user-friendly format for distributing this information to students (Center for Mental Health in Schools, 1997). A sample of such a card is provided in Figure 4.2.

Schools have also found school health fairs to be an effective method of supplying students with these important resources and knowledge. A variety of issues could be addressed in this format by asking interested community agencies to staff a booth with an informed employee who could answer ques-

SIDE ONE		SIDE TWO	
General Services		*Child Abuse / Domestic Violence*	
River City Mental Health	(888) 555-0000	**Violence Prevention Coalition**	(888) 555-7777
123 River Drive, River City			
		Child Abuse Hotline	(888) 555-STOP
XYZ Counseling	(888) 555-1111	**Safety First**	(888) 555-3987
333 Alpha St., River City		444 First St., Rock Town	
Runaway		*Drug / Alcohol*	
A Teen's Place	(888) 555-TEEN	**Oak Tree Dependency Center**	(888) 554-9324
Location is confidential		5423 Palm Ave., River City	
Runaway Hotline	(888) 555-2222		
		Alcoholics Anonymous	(888) 555-9325
Shelters			
River City Women's Shelter	(888) 555-3131	*Family Planning*	
99 Blair Circle, River City		**River City Health Dept.**	(888) 555-4545
		125 River Drive, River City	
Hearts Home	(888) 555-HOME		
		Other Services	
Rape		**River City/Rock City Police Dept.**	Dial 911
Rape Victims Hotline	(888) 555-HELP		

FIGURE 4.2. Sample wallet-sized resource card for students. (It is a good idea to laminate the cards.)

tions and provide brochures and information. Agencies from fields such as drug/alcohol dependency, domestic violence, shelters, nutrition, park district, and after-school clubs could be included. Any agency that would improve the physical and mental health of students could be invited to participate. Most of these agencies are skilled at providing quick, fun, age-appropriate activities regarding their field. Ideally the fair would be offered at two different times—once during the school day for students and once during the evening for parents and students.

In addition to maintaining records on child resources, providing referral information on adult services, such as parenting classes or women's shelters, is not beyond the proper bounds of practice for school-based practitioners. By helping parents to improve their functioning, the child ultimately benefits.

Family

Just as when deciding whether to refer students to community resources or to provide only school-based services, the circumstances of the family should be considered when making a referral to an outside organization. These include the financial situation of the family, its perception of mental health services, the level of interest in receiving services, and other needs, such as transportation or child care. The family's insurance status is an important factor to consider. If the family does not have insurance or the insurance plan does not cover mental health services, most likely the family will be limited to services with a sliding fee scale. If they have insurance that covers mental health, that may open more doors to mental health providers in private practice.

On the other hand, the insurance may pay for services but limit payment to a particular provider, which is common with HMO plans. If the family has a PPO insurance provider, a variety of private practitioners or outpatient mental health services are reimbursed for services, making the selection of providers less limited. Regardless of the type of insurance, school professionals should encourage the family to review their particular policy to determine what type of services are reimbursable and how many sessions are covered.

In addition to the financial resources available to the family, their prior experiences with mental health services appear to affect their likelihood of following through with a referral. A study of women at domestic violence shelters found that mothers who had received counseling in the past were more likely to follow through with a referral for their child than women who had not participated in counseling (Webersinn, Hollinger, & DeLamatre, 1991). Parents' understanding of the benefits of mental health services for children seems to be a prerequisite for follow-through (Webersinn et al., 1991). This makes the discussion of mental health issues with parents another important component of the referral process, as it is likely a key determinant of the effectiveness of the referral (Webersinn et al., 1991).

Child Characteristics

As when deciding whether to provide services at school, the characteristics of the child should play a large part in deciding to whom to refer the child. The type of services the child needs and the nature of the problems the child and family are facing should guide referral decisions. Common sense would lead one to think that a match between client and clinician on race/ethnicity and gender would be important, especially for dealing with such sensitive topics as abuse and neglect. Regardless of the racial match between client and clinician, it is important for the clinician to have an awareness and understanding of other cultures in order to reduce treatment attrition (Wade & Bernstein, 1991). Wade and Bernstein (1991) found that clinicians who had received culture sensitivity training but were not necessarily racially matched with their clients had higher client follow-through rates than clinicians who had not received such training. While racial similarity also contributed to lower attrition rates, culturally sensitive clinicians were recommended when a racial match was not possible (Wade & Bernstein, 1991).

Choosing a referral source can be done with the family. The most important thing to remember is to not merely hand the parent a name and phone number. The Center for Mental Health in Schools (1997) states that the common practice of giving the parent three names and phone numbers to contact is not enough. School-based practitioners have been trained to work effectively with people, to use good communication techniques, and to access data, all of which are skills that can make the referral process successful. They must describe the most appropriate resources to parents and discuss the advantages and limitations of each for meeting the particular needs of the family's situation. It is likely that there will not be an agency that is a perfect fit for the family, but there will be one that best fits each family.

AFTER MAKING A REFERRAL

If the child is going to be receiving services from an outside therapist, there are still ways for staff to support the child within the school setting. If the school is invested in making the referral and intervention effective, once it has been decided where to refer the child for outside services, the school should continue to work with the child and family throughout the referral process. There are three phases of referral follow up: initial case placement, ongoing progress monitoring, and ancillary school services (for children transitioning back to school after a different placement or for those who remain in the school but receive primary therapy from an outside source). The types of tasks suggested in following up on a referral include checking with the family about progress in obtaining services, maintaining a collaborative relationship with the outside therapist, coordinating services with CPS, making placement decisions, creating supervision plans (if necessary), and providing alternative services to the child in addition to the primary therapy.

Initial Case Placement

When following through with the child's family, the school must act only as a supporter. The family, ultimately, unless mandated by CPS, has the right to decide if services will be sought and who will provide those services. Families might appreciate follow-up contact after the referral has been made, because obstacles to receiving services do arise, either from the social service system or from within the family itself. The school staff may suggest or help enlist resources or connections to help the family overcome some of these barriers, such as the problem of affordable transportation.

Progress Monitoring

The relationship between the therapist and the school may be critical in making the limited time the therapist has with the child or family most effective. Ongoing contact with the therapist allows for concerns from the perspective of the school to be shared with the therapist and for the therapist to share recommendations for continued support in the school (Horton, 1996). Legally the school must obtain consent from the legal guardian—or CPS, if the child is a ward of the state—in order to (1) obtain information from outside sources and (2) release information to outside sources. Each release must clearly state the names of the individuals who will be sharing or receiving information (i.e., not simply the names of the organizations), the type of information that will be shared, the client involved, the length of time for which the release will be valid, how the information will be used, the consequences of not giving consent, and how the guardian can revoke consent. Releases must be obtained for each agency with which the school wishes to have contact. The samples shown in Figures 4.3 and 4.4 are only meant to be used as examples, because the guidelines provided by each state and district on these issues may vary.

When thinking about exchanging information, one must balance the need to share information with the need for therapeutic privacy. The therapist most likely will not share every detail of the therapeutic work but instead may provide a general overview of the work that is being done and the progress being made. This brings up another point that should be mentioned. Many schools have the philosophy that the entire school staff is responsible for the welfare of each child. This may lead to a need to revisit privacy and confiden-

CONSENT FOR RELEASE OF INFORMATION

I, _____, give my consent and permission for _____
    (name of parent/guardian)   (name of
_____ at ABC School to release information concerning _____
    professional)   (name of student)
psychological assessment and/or treatment to:

_____.

(name of clinician/mental health provider to receive the information)

The information released may include, but not be limited to, data gained from interview and testing session(s) with ABC School staff as well as the staff's discussions and opinions of this material. The purpose of this release is to:

_____

_____.

(reason for release; usually it is to coordinate services and collaborate on treatment)

The consequences (if any) of not signing this release would be:

_____

_____

This release can be withdrawn at any time by notifying ABC School in writing. This release will expire in one year. I am aware of my right to inspect the information to be released.

_____   _____
Parent or guardian (or student,   Date
if over age 18)

_____   _____
Student (if ages 12–17)   Date

_____   _____
Witness   Date

FIGURE 4.3. Sample consent for release of information.

tiality within the school setting. A good practice for schools to follow is to share information within the school only on a need-to-know basis.

It is also best practice to keep records of each contact with outside agencies, whether it is with the therapist or CPS. The date of the contact, who was contacted, the client discussed, and a description of what was discussed would be useful for planning interventions and documenting what has been done for the child. For successful collaboration, inviting the outside therapist

CONSENT TO OBTAIN INFORMATION

I, _____, give my consent and permission for:
(name of parent or guardian)

_____
(name of clinician/mental health provider who will be sharing the information)
to release the following information concerning _____
(name of student)

to _____ at ABC School: _____
_____.

The purpose of this release is to: _____
_____
(reason for release; usually it is to coordinate services and collaborate on treatment)

The consequences (if any) of not signing this release would be:
_____
_____
(consequences of not signing; usually it is no disclosure/sharing of information)

This release can be withdrawn by me at any time by notifying ABC School in writing. This release will expire in one year. I am aware of my right to inspect the information to be released.

_____   _____
Parent or guardian (or student,   Date
if over age 18)

_____   _____
Student (if ages 12–17)   Date

_____   _____
Witness   Date

FIGURE 4.4. Sample consent to obtain information.

or the CPS representative to multidisciplinary meetings may further facilitate communication.

Ideally, communication should go both ways. The school can offer a great deal of unique information to the outside agency. The school psychologist can offer periodic behavioral observations, psychoeducational evaluation results, and teacher perceptions via checklists and behavioral rating forms. The normative information teachers can provide to special services staff and mental health providers should not be overlooked. A veteran teacher has seen hundreds of students, making his/her knowledge of typical behavior and functioning at a specific grade level unsurpassable. While such information may be helpful to an outside clinician for initial assessment purposes, a school-based perspective may also be important in monitoring treatment progress. The sample letter provided in Figure 4.5 illustrates how school-based practitioners may invite collaboration from a particular outside agency providing a child mental health services.

Ancillary Services

Finally, the school-based practitioner can provide further intervention to the child by either providing (1) ancillary services, such as working on anger management, but not primarily dealing with the maltreatment and/or (2)

Dear colleague:

I have recently referred a student, _____, and his/her family to your agency. I am the school psychologist at _____ School. After consulting with other school staff and the child's family or guardian, we felt that the student's needs could best be met through additional outside services. After examining various options, your organization was thought to be appropriate for this student.

If the child's family or legal guardian has not already contacted you regarding this referral, you should be hearing from them shortly. Attached are copies of all of the necessary releases so that we can exchange information, as needed, about the client.

As you may already know, the school can provide you with various types of information that may be useful in your work with the child or family. Psychoeducational, observational, behavioral, or socioemotional information may be available about this child. In the past, teachers have been very willing to complete behavioral checklists or other types of forms about our students, as well. Please do not hesitate to inquire about any of this information if you believe it could be helpful for your initial assessment and treatment planning, or for ongoing progress monitoring.

Any recommendations you may have for this child in the school setting would be welcomed. If ancillary services are provided within the school, I will contact you in order to avoid duplication of services, integrate our treatment plans, and monitor progress.

The staff at _____ School is very committed to meeting the needs of all students. This being so, we encourage you to contact us with any questions and look forward to collaborating with you.

Sincerely,

School Psychologist

FIGURE 4.5. Sample letter to outside agency inviting collaboration.

creating an environment in which the child can feel comfortable and successful. When providing additional therapy to the child, it is especially recommended that there be ongoing communication with the child's primary therapist so that services are coordinated and do not overlap. The environment
of the school can also be modified through consultations with teachers on
how to support the child in the classroom (see Chapter 6).

A final list of suggested practices is included in Figure 4.6 as a quick reference for the entire referral process.

DOs:

Check with the families prior to choosing a referral source; their values and opinions are
valuable in selecting the best options.

Examine the various organizations before referring a family; match the needs of the client
with what the agency has to offer.

Update records of community resources on a regular basis.

Make the information readily available to students and parents; consider finding a location in which the information can be used anonymously, without having to make a formal
appointment.

Consider holding a health fair with other local schools; invite various health and mental
health providers; consider having it during school hours and a time for parents to attend
after school.

Keep adult referral information for parents who may need assistance (i.e., information on
shelters, parenting groups, adult mental health providers).

Check on waiting lists, sliding fee scales, and insurance details before making a referral.

Encourage families to examine their insurance coverage before choosing a referral source.

Follow through with families. Offer to let them call the agency for the first time with you;
ask if any additional services are needed; check on how satisfied the family/child is with
the services.

With permission, keep open communication between the family, the school, and the community agency.

Foster collaborative relationships with community service providers; join relevant task
forces and organizations.

Offer ancillary services, such as anger management or groups for children going through
divorce.

DON'Ts:

Handing the name and phone number of a referral source to a family is not sufficient.

Don't assume the family's values regarding mental health services are the same as yours or
the school's.

Don't try to do it all yourself; collaborate with other school professionals, the family, and
outside resources, when appropriate.

FIGURE 4.6. Referral tips.

CONCLUSION

Deciding which children should be served in the school setting and which should be referred to outside services can be an overwhelming process. Moreover, an often overlooked component of this process is how to make an effective referral to an outside agency. Professional training in the referral process is often not provided, so the procedures implemented may be inadequate for truly meeting the needs of maltreated children. The goal of an effective referral should be to increase the likelihood of the family's following through with the referral and the student's receiving efficacious treatment. Client follow-through for services is very important, especially when working with families facing abuse and/or neglect issues; without support from the person making the referral, follow-through is unlikely to occur for these families. They often face numerous stressors and emotional factors, such as guilt or shame, that may inhibit follow-through. For some families, merely handing them a slip of paper with a phone number on it might be enough for the contact to be made; this practice, however, is not recommended even for that family. By working with the family to find treatment and with the service provider to coordinate services, the school practitioner will more likely enable families to find satisfying services and to continue participation in the services. Most importantly, the child will feel supported.

CHAPTER 5

School-Based Mental Health Services for Victims of Child Maltreatment

♦

Once it is determined that the school may have a role in providing mental health interventions for children and adolescents who have been abused, there are a variety of options to consider. Many students with a history of abuse may benefit from general mental health treatments. Some may best be treated in groups specifically for children who have been abused. Finally, abuse-focused counseling might be provided to certain children on a one-to-one basis.

GENERAL MENTAL HEALTH INTERVENTIONS

Children with histories of abuse may benefit from a number of services already provided by the schools. For example, groups for children with anxiety or depression may be helpful to many children who have internalized the effects of abuse. Anger control groups might include abused children who have externalized their distress. Instruction in social skills, assertiveness training, affective education—virtually any general group provided by schools may be appropriate for some children have been abused, as long as the topic is matched to their particular symptoms. In many cases it may be left up to the child to decide whether or not to disclose what contributed to the development of anxiety or the feelings of rage; irrespective of that consideration, developing coping strategies and having a positive safe experience with peers are usually helpful therapeutic treatments.

In addition to including children who have been abused in groups that match their symptoms, it may be helpful to consider including these students in groups focused on particular situations or life stressors that pertain to their world. For example, a group for children who have recently moved might be particularly helpful. Children who are maltreated move twice as frequently as their cohorts, resulting in lower test scores, lower grades, and increased likelihood of repeating grades (Eckenrode, Rowe, Laird, & Brathwaite, 1995). Such findings persist even when related variables such as public assistance status are controlled for statistically. It has been speculated that moves may have such a negative effect on the school performance of children who have been maltreated because (1) their social isolation increases as they lose friends, neighbors, teachers, and classmates; (2) they are emotionally affected by the moves and this, in turn, affects learning; (3) there are likely differences between curricula and teacher expectations between old and new schools; and (4) others in the family (parents and siblings) are also likely stressed by the move, so the home environment produces additional stressors for the child (Eckenrode et al., 1995).

As the divorce literature has well documented, it is often these secondary stressors that mediate a child's emotional outcome. Thus, addressing these issues, such as moving, may be quite useful. Additional possibilities might include children whose parents are divorced or divorcing or going through other family changes. Again, children will also likely benefit from seeing that they are not alone and by having additional positive social connections.

ABUSE-SPECIFIC INTERVENTIONS

Some school practitioners, depending on the answers to questions raised earlier, are willing and able to provide abuse-specific interventions, either in group or individual sessions with students. Before developing such a program of therapy, it is appropriate to consider the relevant professional literature regarding what has been documented as effective.

What Works?

A decade ago one of the authors was meeting with the clinical director of a social service agency, discussing an upcoming training session regarding the treatment of abused children. In this meeting he was clarifying what he had hoped his clinical staff would learn. " I want you to talk to them about what works," he said. Thinking about the infancy of the field and the lack of systematic program evaluations, the author immediately replied, "Honestly, we don't really know." Instantly the clinical director retorted, "Don't tell them that!" It is not so much that he was looking for a dishonest presentation as it was that he was pointing out the dilemma. Whether or not a standard of academic rigor had been met in the field, these clinicians would be facing children who have been abused today. These clinicians could not wait for definitive answers. They needed the author's best, hopefully somewhat informed, opinion *today*. They needed suggestions. These clinicians needed to hear about theories that could help them understand the impact of their clients' abuse experience and thereby inform their treatment. These clinicians needed to hear what others were doing, especially if programs seemed successful (even if evidence of some success was based on case studies, small samples, or program evaluations without matched control groups). They needed answers, not to be told there are none.

Unfortunately, nearly a decade later, the situation has not changed as much as many had hoped. Reviewing the state of the field, Saunders and Williams (1996) report that, while "treatment for abused children is viewed as appropriate, necessary, and even mandatory by most mental health professionals and child advocates . . . scientific knowledge about the outcome of treatment for abused children lags far behind the clinical literature, the clinical practice, and the high volume of services being delivered" (p. 293).

School professionals, however, are faced with numerous children in need of services today. Fortunately, just as there was enough information then to present an in-service training session to the clinical staff, there is some—in fact, substantially more—relevant information available today. Theories have been refined, model programs have been described, and the scientific knowledge has increased somewhat. In fact, Saunders and Williams's somewhat bleak comment quoted above was in an introduction to a special issue of *Child Maltreatment* that included three outcome studies that they recognized as "important steps toward correcting this deficit in empirical, research-based knowledge about treatment of abused children" (p. 293). A number of additional outcome studies have been published since that November 1996 issue. Thus, there are still many unknowns, but the outlook is improving. Valuable theoretical models have been described. Important treatment goals and approaches have been discussed. Treatment manuals of model programs are being made available. Following is a review of each of those areas.

Theoretical Perspectives

Numerous theoretical perspectives have been offered as ways of understanding the effects of maltreatment and conceptualizing the needed treatment. Certainly, many of these perspectives have an extensive base of related research; therefore, programs built on these, while perhaps not yet the subject of systematic outcome research, have solid grounding. While many of the individual perspectives have considerable value, a thorough review of each is beyond the scope of this book; however, several of them are briefly summarized in Chapter 6.

One recent model (1995), an "integrated contextual model," has been proposed by Friedrich in his book *Psychotherapy with Sexually Abused Boys* (and elsewhere, e.g., Friedrich, 1996) and is worthy of some special attention. This model, which certainly applies to children of both genders victimized by any form of maltreatment, is based on solid empirical evidence and integrates three important theories: attachment theory, behavioral and emotional regulation, and self-perception/development. These three theories, Friedrich argues, make critical contributions to our understanding of the effects of child abuse and our thinking regarding effective treatment.

Attachment is a complex theory and area of research (Friedrich, 1995). In brief, the theory suggests that closeness—a bond—to a caregiver is critical to healthy development (Bowlby, 1982). "A child needs to be lovingly attached to a reliable parental figure." In fact, "this need is a primary motivating force in human life" (Karen, 1994, p. 441). Parents, ideally, provide a "secure base" that enables a child to feel safe and later able to explore the world. Another tenet of the theory is the concept of the internal working model, the idea that these primary attachment relationships form a child's understanding of his/her own role in relationships (Am I worthy? lovable?) and others' roles in relationships (Are people there for me? Will I be cared for?), which guides his/her expectations and behavior in future relationships. This internal working model has both cognitive and affective components and results in styles of attachment.

Children, according to this conceptual literature and empirical research, will develop a secure or insecure attachment style. Those with secure attachments are likely to have the most optimal outcomes. Those with insecure attachments may develop resistant/ambivalent, avoidant, or disorganized patterns in their relationships with the caregivers and others later in life. Not surprisingly, child abuse and neglect interfere with the development of secure attachments. In fact, as many as 85% of maltreated children have insecure attachments (Carlson, Cicchetti, Barnett, & Braunwald, 1989; Karen, 1994). A secure base has simply not been established. Factors such as fear, unresolved trauma, rejection, and parent–child role reversal interfere with the ability to attach securely (Alexander, 1992).

The implications of the attachment perspective in working with abused children are many. First, clinicians working with children with insecure attachments must be especially careful to be accepting of the child. Clinicians must very intentionally work to form a sense of safety and a therapeutic alliance. Attachments not only with the therapist but also with the primary caregivers should be supported. Finally, the therapist working from this perspective seeks to "chip away" at the distorted internal working model so that the child may begin to believe "I am worthy of love" and "People will be there for me" (Friedrich, 1995).

The second component of Friedrich's model, a dysregulation perspective, describes trauma, particularly in children, as overwhelming to the individual, beyond his/her ability to understand or cope. "When the usual means of dealing with experience are not useful, the person becomes overwhelmed and disorganized. The resulting, dysregulating impact of trauma occurs along a range of effects, including neurophysiological, behavioral, and cognitive" (Friedrich, 1995, p. 98). Dysregulation, put simply, is the reaction to being faced with "too much too soon."

The field is just beginning to understand the neuropsychological impact of trauma. It is increasingly clear, however, that trauma, particularly prolonged stress in young children, has a physiological impact on brain development. A child's dysregulated central nervous system may have an impact on numerous areas of functioning, such as affect, anxiety, arousal, impulse control, memory, and cognition. Behaviorally, the effects of dysregulation, Friedrich argues (1995) may be seen in sleep disorders, PTSD, ADHD, affective lability, suicidality, compulsive behaviors, explosive outbursts, dissociative disorders, and sexually reactive behavior. Cognitively, dysregulation may show itself in persistent, intrusive, hopeless thoughts, memory disturbance, and academic difficulty.

A dysregulation perspective would suggest that therapy should be structured and predictable (to help reduce anxiety). Additionally, this point of view would suggest that children be taught self-soothing tension-reduction skills and other coping techniques to begin to understand and regulate their own affect, cognitions, and behaviors (Friedrich, 1995).

Finally, self theory is the third component that Friedrich includes in his integrated contextual model. According to this theory (per Kegan, 1982, and others) children are "meaning-making individuals" who are constantly working to understand who they are in relation to other persons. Certainly child maltreatment can interfere with the development of a healthy sense of self. Victims may begin to believe the cognitive distortions of their perpetrators: "You're no good. You deserve this. You are sick. You asked for it" (Burton & Rasmussen, 1998). Object relations theory describes the process as the development of the internalized "bad object," an increasing sense of oneself as the bad, abusive perpetrator (Friedrich, 1995).

Self theory would argue that therapy should be responsive to children's needs to develop healthier ways to identify their feelings, learn to externalize their problems, change inappropriate cognitions, develop competencies, and develop a more positive view of the self (Friedrich, 1995). The relationship context of therapy provides them the opportunity to experience acceptance, affirmation, and a positive view of self in relationship with a significant other.

While the integrated contextual model is comprehensive, combining a variety of the most critical perspectives, two others are worth noting here: the social information-processing model and cognitive-behavioral theory.

The social information-processing model has received special attention from the maltreatment field (e.g., O'Donohue & Rudman, 1999; Price & Landsverk, 1998). Simply put, the model suggests that the way in which a child processes social information will directly influence his/her psychosocial functioning (Crick & Dodge, 1996). Early family experiences (caregiving experience, attachment, or abuse) in concert with biologically based capabilities result in a child's knowledge and feelings about him/herself and others (Dodge, Pettit, Bates, & Valente, 1995). A child processes current social information in this light. So, not surprisingly, an abused child is more likely to interpret current situations negatively, or with a "hostile attribution bias." A neutral situation, such as a classmate knocking a book off of a student's desk, is more likely to be interpreted by an abused child as a deliberate affront and reacted to accordingly. Additionally, he/she may have distorted cognitions about the legitimacy of retaliation and aggression (e.g., "Hey, he knocked my book over—I was just getting him back.") and immunity from consequences (e.g., "Me? Go to the principal's office? Why? I was just doin' what I had to do") (Feindler, 1991). The social information-processing model does not suggest that all abused children will develop these patterns or that they cannot be altered. In fact, social information-processing variables have been found to mediate the relationship between physical abuse and aggressive behavior (Dodge et al., 1995), and a number of approaches to changing the cognitions have been discussed.

Certainly, this theory suggests steps for intervention, particularly the use of cognitive restructuring to address the need to consider other social cues, other possible attributions of others' intentions, and the generation of more appropriate responses (Feindler, 1991).

Social informational-processing perspectives and techniques are closely related to the broader cognitive-behavioral theory, which assumes that "behavioral events, associated anticipatory expectations and post event attributions, ongoing cognitive information processing, and emotional states combine to influence behavior change" (Kendall, 1991, p. 3). Put simply, this theory emphasizes the interactional nature of thoughts, feelings, and behavior. Meichenbaum (1997), among others, has applied this view to the treatment of victims of child abuse, particularly those with PTSD.

The applications are quite straightforward. Acting in the roles of consultant, diagnostician, and educator/coach, a cognitive-behavioral therapist uses "active, performance-based procedures as well as cognitive interventions to produce changes in thinking, feeling, and behavior" (Kendall, 1991) when assisting child or adolescent clients with a history of child maltreatment. Common techniques used include affective education, cognitive restructuring techniques, and skills training, which—particularly for children—are integrated into a game format.

Treatment Goals

While the integrated contextual model, the social information-processing model, and cognitive-behavioral theory are applicable to understanding many victims of child maltreatment and have direct implications for their treatment, case planning must be individualized. There is no simple recipe or formula that will be suitable for the school professional to use with every child or group of children who have experienced child maltreatment. Abuse is a historical event, not a diagnosis, so the treatment needs and therapeutic goals will vary tremendously (Horton & Cruise, 1997b). "First and foremost, it is urgent to view each child's experience as unique" (Gil, 1991, p. 38).

Individualized multimethod, multi-informant assessment using child, parent, and teacher interviews (see Salter, 1988) and general instruments (e.g., the Children's Depression Inventory, the Child Behavior Checklist), as well as abuse-specific measures (e.g., the Trauma Symptom Checklist for Children, the Children's Sexual Behavior Inventory), is critical. While a number of specific programs and additional resources that may be helpful to consider are mentioned throughout this text, it is critical that school psychologists, social workers, or counselors create the program to best meet the needs of their particular student clients.

There are, however, certain common goals and treatment considerations that apply to work with many clients with a history of abuse. In the context of a therapeutic relationship, the treatment of children who have been abused typically needs to address the affective, cognitive, behavioral, and social effects of the maltreatment experience.

Therapeutic Relationship

When working with children or adolescents with a history of abuse or neglect, the importance of the therapeutic relationship cannot be overemphasized. In her classic work *Trauma and Recovery*, Herman makes the point emphatically: "Recovery can take place only in the context of relationships; it cannot occur in isolation." She notes that maltreatment damages the basic capacities for trust, autonomy, initiative, competence, identity, and intimacy. "Just as these capabilities are originally formed in relationships with other people, they must be reformed in such relationships" (Herman, 1992, p. 133). Similarly, Gil has pointed out that "because abuse is interactional," children who have been victimized can "profit from an opportunity to experience a safe, appropriate, and rewarding interaction with a trusted other" (Gil, 1991, p. 53).

Clearly, then, the relationship aspect seems central to abuse-focused therapy. School-based clinicians must consider a number of aspects involved in developing a positive therapeutic relationship.

1. The clinician's attitude should be positive and engaging. While therapy may appropriately focus on abuse, this does not imply that the counselor should have a cold, clinical focus on pathology (Briere, 1992).

2. The experience must be nonintrusive. Children who have been abused have had their boundaries violated. "Because physical and sexual abuse are intrusive acts, the clinician's interventions should be non-intrusive, allowing the child ample physical and emotional space" (Gil, 1991, p. 59).

3. Boundaries need to be clear. Children who have grown up in chaotic families especially need to know the plans, rules, and expectations. How often and how long will the sessions be? What is expected of the child? Are there rules? Without being rigid, a sense of structure creates predictability and a sense of safety.

4. The child must feel safe. A child will not begin to explore and process traumatic material if he/she does not feel safe. It is important to recognize it is not just actual safety (e.g., you know you will not hurt the child, will not violate confidentiality) but that the child has the perception of safety (Salter, 1988). If the child seems unsettled, or unwilling to open up, it may be important to consider what, from his/her point of view, still seems unsafe.

5. The child must be given choices. Abuse frequently creates a "profound experience of helplessness" (Salter, 1988, p. 215). Thus, empowering a child to have choices available at his/her developmental level is a critical principle of recovery (Herman, 1992).

The experience of a relationship with the features just described not only provides the base to do the needed therapeutic work, but also the relationship in itself is therapeutic. A healthy therapist–child relationship provides the opportunity to create a "new map of interpersonal relationships." A therapeutic relationship also contributes by creating a positive and meaningful experience in case the need arises for additional therapy later (Friedrich, 1990).

Affective Component

In the context of a therapeutic relationship, a child can begin to express, explore, and ventilate affect, including anxiety, frustration, rage, or anger, toward the offender, and grief for all that has been lost (Brassard & Gelardo, 1987; Salter, 1988; Wheeler & Berliner, 1988). Children and adolescents may need to learn to recognize their own feelings of emotional pain, guilt, anger, and ambivalence (Salter, 1988). For some, this is a new experience, as they have felt "numb" for so long.

While it is important to encourage affective experience and exploration, it is also important to help children and adolescents not become overwhelmed. Thus, affect regulation skills are important to develop (Briere,

1992; Kendall et al., 1991). Children and adolescents may need assistance in specific coping techniques to handle overwhelming emotions outside of therapy. For example, relaxation techniques may be used to assist children in reducing anxiety. Bedtime rituals may be helpful with night terrors and insomnia (Wheeler & Berliner, 1988).

Affect regulation is also taught experientially in the therapy session. "The pace and focus of psychotherapy rests not only on the client's relative ability to tolerate additional stress at any given point in time, but also on the inherent structure of the session" (Briere, 1992, p. 103). The following phases are important in each session:

- Begin with low intensity: "So, how was your weekend? How are things going in Mrs. Williams's class?"
- Build to a peak around midsession: "Last time, you mentioned there were some scary things that used to happen when your uncle lived with you. . . ."
- Return to baseline by the end: "OK, I guess it is about time to get you back to class. You have PE, next, right? What sports do you enjoy. . . ."

The middle phase of each session has been described as the "therapeutic window," the opportunity to focus on the most intensive issues (Briere, 1992). While the three phases of the session will generally remain in the same order, the amount of time spent in each will change. Initially, there may be quite a bit of time "warming up" and "winding down," with limited time being spent in the middle phase. The "therapeutic window" is brief at first. As the therapeutic relationship continues, however, the beginning and ending phases can become shorter and the "therapeutic window" will become the majority of the session.

The final, wind down, or "return to baseline" phase may remain quite important, particularly in a school setting, as the client will be returning to class to face peers and teachers. Talking about a traumatic memory two minutes before the client will be sitting in algebra class is certainly not a sensitive, or wise therapeutic move; a longer transition is required.

There are occasions in which clients come to the session already upset, jumping right into the "therapeutic window." A teacher may bring a child, or send an adolescent, to the counseling office because the student was distressed and crying in class. In these instances, there is "no reasonable way to avoid immediately high levels of painful affect"; however, these situations "require serious attention to provide the client with some level of de-arousal before the end of the session" (Briere, 1992, p. 103).

Intensity control is especially crucial in reducing after-session "acting out." If a high school counselor learns that an adolescent client is engaging in self-mutilation ("cutting") or drug or alcohol use immediately after the counseling sessions, pause should be taken. It is quite likely that these behaviors are the adolescent's use of "tension-reduction devices to deal with therapy-restimulated abuse trauma" (Briere, 1992, pp. 103–104). A wise counselor, then, shortens the "therapeutic window," bringing the tension down sooner, allowing the student to have a sense of closure and "reconstitute defenses" before leaving the session. The student then will hopefully have less need for later, more drastic, measures to reduce tension.

Much of the important affective issues dealt with in the "therapeutic window" relate to exploring, reprocessing, and desensitization of painful memories. Thus, the cognitive aspects also become important (Briere, 1992).

Cognitive Component

In addition to expressing, processing, and learning to modulate their emotions, children who have been maltreated must learn to make sense of what has happened to them. Distorted, hurtful thinking patterns often result from abusive experiences. While each child's experience is unique, the following cognitions are common among children who are being abused (Briere, 1992, p. 28):

1. "I am being hurt, emotionally or physically, by a parent or other trusted adult."
2. "Based on how I think about the world thus far, this injury can only be due to one of two things: Either I am bad or my parent is bad" (the abuse dichotomy).
3. "I have been taught by other adults, either at home or in school, that parents are always right, and always do things for your own good (any other alternative is very frightening). When they occasionally hurt you, it is for your own good, because you have been bad. This is called punishment."
4. "Therefore, it must be my fault that I am being hurt, just as my parent says. This must be punishment. I must deserve this."
5. "Therefore, I am as bad as whatever is done to me (the punishment must fit the crime: anything else suggests parental badness, which I have rejected). I am bad because I have been hurt. I have been hurt because I am bad."
6. "I am hurt quite often and/or quite deeply; therefore I must be very bad."

Clearly, such cognitive distortions are understandable yet destructive. Children must learn to process and make sense of the trauma (Gil, 1991). They must learn to understand the abuse experience differently and to view themselves differently (Deblinger & Heflin, 1996; Friedrich, 1990).

First, victims of child maltreatment must make new meaning of their abuse experience (Friedrich, 1990). In particular, they must learn to alter their attribution of responsibility for the abuse. Frequently, because of what perpetrators or significant others have said or implied, victims feel responsible or to blame for what has occurred (Hindman, 1999). Information about abuse (e.g., "It is a crime") and offenders ("They made a very wrong choice") presented in a developmentally appropriate way, combined with repeated opportunities to specifically examine and correct distorted cognitions, may be important in helping victims "get off the hook" and begin to gain a restored sense of self-efficacy (Salter, 1988; Wheeler & Berliner, 1988).

Children and adolescents who have been victimized also frequently have distorted, destructive thoughts about themselves that need to be addressed. Children may feel as though they are the "only ones" that have had such an experience. They may feel bad, dirty, or evil because of it. Additionally, victims may feel "crazy" due to their PTSD symptoms. Normalization is, therefore, an important activity. Many children may seem relieved too when the therapist explains that they are not the only victims—that, unfortunately, many children have been abused. Groups or books on the subject seem to illustrate that point even more poignantly ("Wow, there really are others like me, who have been through things that I have been through! And I don't think badly of them"). Additionally, symptoms can be normalized and explained as having served previous functions (Briere, 1992). "Lots of children have those feelings. It was good, when you were living with your father, to be "extra on guard" all of the time, because that helped you know when to try to hide. Now that you are living in a safe place, you will just have to teach yourself that it is OK to relax now." Finally, it is critical to enhance accurate perceptions of the self (Friedrich, 1990). Therapists should use every opportunity to intervene in any self-derogation and to help children think of themselves as more than a victim (Briere, 1992; Friedrich, 1990).

Thus, various cognitive techniques can be used to gently challenge previous interpretations and provide healthier ways of thinking. Less distorted cognitions can lead to less distressed, happier affective states (Kendall et al., 1991). Additionally, cognitive interventions are also important as a precedent for behavioral interventions (Garbarino, 1987). As long as a child thinks "I must be bad," he/she has little motivation to learn to "act good." A restructured cognitive map may allow the child to incorporate new behaviors.

Behavioral and Social Components

Addressing behavior problems and enhancing the child's prosocial repertoire are important goals for many children who have been maltreated (Garbarino, 1987; Kolko, 1992). Children who have been abused and neglected may have overwhelming emotions and distorted cognitions, which contribute to the development of behavioral and social difficulties. Further, many mal-treated children have had numerous inappropriate antisocial role models (Kolko, 1992). Therefore, while not likely effective or appropriate by them-selves, behavioral interventions, when integrated with other approaches, are relevant in dealing with maltreated, traumatized children, largely because they help to build up one's social competence (Garbarino, 1987).

Specific behavior goals and techniques will vary, depending on the child's current functioning (Friedrich, 1990). For some, anger management skills training may be imperative due to problems with impulsive and/or ag-gressive behavior (Haskett & Kistner, 1991; Lewis, 1992). For other clients, such social skills as assertiveness, empathy building, or other communication training may be important (Lewis, 1992; Salter, 1988). Bloomquist's (1996) *Skills Training for Children with Behavior Disorders: A Parent and Therapist Guidebook* offers numerous relevant tools.

Abuse-Specific Symptomatology

In addition to addressing general emotional, cognitive, and behavioral issues that may be present in the aftermath of child maltreatment, therapists work-ing with children and adolescents who have been abused and neglected must be prepared to address abuse-specific symptomatology.

PTSD

Children and adolescents may need assistance in understanding a variety of their PTSD symptoms (e.g., nightmares, flashbacks), subject as they are to worries that nobody feels as they do or that they may be "going crazy." Books, handouts, or materials that demonstrate that other children have had similar feelings, that the experience actually does makes sense, and there are steps they can take to decrease symptoms over time may be encouraging. One such example is the "PTSD Workbook" in Cunningham and MacFar-lane's (1996) *When Children Abuse*. In this booklet children receive a develop-mentally sensitive explanation (e.g., while the actual PTSD terminology is explained in child-oriented language, the authors also encourage child clients to think of PTSD as standing for "Pretty Tough Stuff, Dude." Specific sug-gestions are offered, and children are encouraged to write and draw about their experience throughout.

Dissociation

One specific PTSD or child maltreatment symptom that deserves special at-tention is dissociation. Herman (1992) describes why this is a particularly common phenomenon among those who have survived abuse: "The child victim prefers to believe that the abuse did not occur. In the service of this wish, she tries to keep the secret from herself. The means she has at her disposal are frank denial, voluntary suppression of thoughts, and a legion of dissociative reactions. The capacity for induced trance or dissociative states, normally high in school-age children, is developed to a fine art" (p. 102).

While dissociation served an important function during the abuse, the symptom may be interfering with a child's current functioning. For example, if a child, without intending to, reverts to a "trance-like" state whenever he/she becomes anxious, this could cause difficulty in social or academic situations. Additionally, there is increasing evidence that a long-term pattern of extensive dissociation is not without costs and may lead to prolonged PTSD and extensive somatic symptoms that persist for years (Herman, 1992).

The following steps have been recommended for directly addressing dissociation (Gil, 1992):

1. Develop a language: "Let's call this your 'spacing out.' "
2. Help determine dissociative sequencing: "You say this happens when you have to give a speech, and you become afraid."
3. Explain it as adaptive: "You had a lot of scary things happen to you when you were younger. It's good that you had some way to escape, even if it was in your mind."
4. Understand precipitants: "So this spacing out happens any time you get nervous or anxious."
5. Address the troublesome emotion: "Do you know what anxiety is and where you feel it in your body? Do you remember feeling anxious when the secret touching started?"
6. Give an alternative to the flight response: "I'm going to teach you some other choices of good things to do when you feel anxious, sort of like different tools to put in your tool chest. That way, if there is a time when you feel anxious, but it is not a good situation to use the 'space out' tool, you can use one of these other tools."

Sexual Behavior Problems

Another abuse-specific behavior that school-based practitioners should have some familiarity with is sexual behavior problems. In their recent review of sexual abuse treatment outcome studies, Finkelhor & Berliner (1995) note that sexual behavior problems are among the most difficult symptoms to extinguish. A thorough review of the treatment of these issues is beyond the scope of this volume and, in fact, has been the sole subject of several other books (see, e.g., Araji, 1997; Gil & Johnson, 1993; Ryan & Lane, 1997a). Such complete coverage may not be necessary for most school practitioners.

School-based clinicians will not typically be the primary therapist treating children for their severe sexual behavior problems. They may, however, serve a supportive role at school in those cases, or they might be involved in less severe situations. Thus, it may be helpful to have some basic information and some sense of relevant resources.

Treatment curricula worthy of consideration for those working with young children include Cunningham and MacFarlane's (1996) *Children Who Abuse: Group Treatment Strategies for Children with Impulse Control Problems*, Johnson's (1995) *Treatment Exercises for Child Abuse Victims and Children with Sexual Behavior Problems*, Burton and Rasmussen's (1998) *Treating Children with Sexually Abusive Behavior Problems*, and Kahn's (1999) *Roadmaps to Recovery: A Guided Workbook for Young People in Treatment.*

These guides provide a variety of exercises to address such issues as self-esteem, anger management, and anxiety control. Sexual victimization as well as perpetration concerns are also a focus. In general, young children with sexual behavior problems should be treated primarily as victims "compassionately and hopefully . . . by thinking about them as developing organisms who are also the victims of some sort of maltreatment, most often sexual" (Friedrich, 1993, p. x). At the same time, deviant sexual behavior should not be minimized or dismissed but taken seriously as "for children who have been victimized and those who have not, sexual behavior problems in childhood are the behaviors most logically associated with the development of offending behavior in adolescence and adulthood" (Berliner & Rawlings, 1991, p. 3). A balanced position with most children with sexual behavior problems, therefore, does not minimize or avoid the concerning behaviors, but treats the victimization issues first before addressing "perpetration concerns." "Remember how we talked about how when your cousin got you involved in the secret touching? You felt so confused and hurt. Well, when you started touching that kindergarten boy on the bus, I think he felt confused and hurt, too. I want to help you learn to make different choices, because the hurting has to stop."

For older students, adolescents with more long-established patterns, matters should be taken even more seriously. Clinically, some of these students might be developing more entrenched or more predatory behaviors and becoming more like adult sex offenders. Thus, their cases often involve law enforcement officers or probation officers, as well as outside clinicians. In these cases, school professionals are even less likely to be the appropriate primary clinicians. Again, though, it may be helpful to have some familiarity with common treatment approaches and issues to provide a supportive role at school. Two of the most commonly used treatment guides for this age group are Kahn's (1996) *Pathways: A Guided Workbook for Youth Beginning Treatment* and Steen's (1997) *The Relapse Prevention Workbook for Youth in Treatment.*

Cutting and Other Self-Injurious Behaviors

A phenomenon increasingly being observed among adolescents, including in high school settings, is a pattern of intentional self-injurious behavior, most notably "cutting." Different than similar gestures with suicidal intentions, these cuts (or in some cases other behaviors such as burning or head banging) serve a different purpose, one that is not easily understood by school personnel—or clinicians for that matter.

A variety of explanations have been offered for the behavior, which is too common among those who have survived abuse. Some survivors describe it as a way to externalize the pain: "I can't stand this pain I feel inside, so I'll get distracted by pain outside." Others describe it as means of proving one's existence: "I just felt so dead inside, like wood or something. If I'm bleeding, at least there is proof I am alive."

Briere (1992) describes the behavior as an effort to reduce tension. Since those who grow up in neglectful or abusive families have not learned to regulate affect well, and since there is overwhelming emotion in response to the maltreatment, the survivor is in a predicament: there is great desire to "turn off the pain" and yet "no way" to do that. Thus, paradoxically, self-injurious behaviors are often the result of a desperate effort to get relief.

Given the serious distress and lack of coping resources that may be evident in adolescents demonstrating this behavior, simply forbidding it, or asking a student to "promise not to" do this anymore, may not be effective. Such directions may have some impact on a survivor's "copycat" friends who have been imitating the behavior at school for the sake of attention, but for those with more intense pain and the least resources, longer-term interventions will be required. It is not until the student has learned to regulate affect and cope with distress that he/she will be ready to completely give up such behaviors. Treatment manuals such as Linehan's (1993) *Skills Training Manual for Treating Borderline Personality Disorder* offer specific assistance in this regard. Linehan's book, for example, has two especially relevant chapters regarding emotional regulation and distress tolerance, with handouts and homework sheets very appropriate for adolescents.

Thus, treatment of children and adolescents who have been maltreated should address the affective, cognitive, behavioral and social, and abuse-specific symptoms that are present.

Stages of Therapy

Herman (1992), in her review of the literature of the treatment of survivors of varied types of trauma, noted a pattern. While various authors might use slightly different language, and issues are admittedly complex, there were typically three phases of therapy noted: safety, remembrance and mourning, and reconnection. While the order that victims of trauma seem to go through in their recovery seems consistent, the amount of time needed for each phase varies dramatically.

In the *safety* phase, the client establishes a secure base, a safety net of sorts, before beginning some difficult work. This certainly includes establishing the safe therapeutic relationship with the counselor but is broader than that. Developing a social support network is also important. For children and adolescents, this may mean ensuring some stability and support from home. If there is none, young clients may not be in a position to do other abuse-focused work. The foundation may feel too "shaky." While a counselor may provide some general support and some initial work, young clients may wait until they are significantly older to more fully explore their abuse issues. The length of the safety phase may vary dramatically. For children and adolescents who have a secure base at home, have a number of friends, and have had generally positive relationships, safety is very quickly established. A student, for example, who has generally had a safe, healthy family life but was abused by someone outside the family such as a coach may fairly readily move through the safety phase. Another who was abused for years by her father, has an unsupportive mother, and has few friends may stay in the safety phase for a while longer.

Remembrance and mourning is the abuse-focused part of the therapy. It is the time to focus on what maltreatment occurred and what related losses have been exacted. Exploring and correcting the affective, cognitive, behavioral and social, and abuse-specific symptoms also occurs during this phase.

Finally, the *reconnection* phase involves moving forward and getting on with life. Important aspects of this involve helping students see themselves as "more than a victim" and as entitled to a positive future. If their social lives have never been properly established, or have been interrupted, helping the student get (re)involved with normal, age-appropriate activities, clubs, and sports may be important.

After the primary three phases of abuse-focused therapy are successfully completed, it is time for termination. As with any counseling or therapy, this time should be handled carefully; however, with clients who have been abused it is especially important to be sensitive since an end to the counseling relationship may restimulate the trauma, loss, and abandonment (Briere, 1992). A few factors can make a big difference in making the termination more therapeutic.

1. *Give advanced notice.* It is important to give clients plenty of advanced notice in a developmentally appropriate way. For younger children, for example, it may be important to look at a simple calendar and see that we will have "four more Wednesdays" to see each other. Older clients, even seniors in high school, also need time to adjust to the idea.

2. *Reflect/compliment.* The school-based therapist should ensure that the child or adolescent client understands that the end of counseling is not a rejection but evidence of their progress. "You have grown so much. When you first came, right after you told about the secret touching going on at your house, you were so upset all of the time. I remember, it was very hard to for you to talk to any grown-ups or play with kids. Now, in here, you talk a lot with me. I see you visiting with your teacher and playing with classmates on the playground. Looks like you are having a lot of fun."

3. *Affirm.* In addition to being complimentary about the child's progress, it is important to affirm your relationship with and the personal qualities of the child. "I enjoyed working with you. You are a very creative, sensitive girl." "You are a fun, energetic boy with great ideas. I won't forget you." A child who has been maltreated has had multiple experiences that damaged his/her sense of self and threw into question the value of personal relationships. While hopefully these issues have been addressed throughout the therapy, reaffirming the child and your relationship is a nice way to wrap up.

4. *Cast a vision.* Finally, it may be useful to help the child imagine a continued, positive future. For young children, props such as "magic" binoculars can make this a fun activity. "I see you, in the future; you are still happy, and making more and more friends. When you get upset, you handle it safely," and so on. For older adolescents, this may be a particularly important activity as well. "When you go off to college next year, I can imagine you really enjoying your newfound freedom. Sometimes college life can be stressful, especially around finals time—or when things go wrong. Given that you now know healthier ways to handle upsetting feelings, I can see you making wise choices, not the ones that cause you more pain in the end. I don't know what major you will choose, but I can see you in a "people" field because you are an insightful, caring, and sensitive person. Drop me a note someday and let me know."

Group Treatment

While much of the foregoing discussion addressed individual counseling—which by itself may be effective for many children who have been maltreated—group therapy is a frequently recommended supplement or alternative (Salter, 1988). Group treatment has a number of advantages, including the following:

1. Groups help to reduce isolation (Salter, 1988). Children often feel that they are the "only one" with such a secret. At the closing session of a group for sexually abused adolescents conducted by one of the authors in a high school setting, when asked to reflect on what the best part of group was, many of the students noted that it was learning that others had had similar experiences that was especially valuable.

2. Groups can help address the "damaged goods syndrome." As children and adolescents have the experience of getting to know others who have been abused, and finding out that others are nice, attractive, smart, funny, and have other positive attributes, students may be able to begin to decrease self-loathing and develop more self-respect. While therapists and others can tell children that there is "nothing wrong with you," allowing clients to make their own judgments about fellow students with similar histories is much more powerful.

3. In group treatment, children have an opportunity to meet their peers and in a safe environment develop connections that extend beyond the group, to the classroom, playground, and other social contexts. For children who have been isolated, this is especially important.

4. Groups provide the opportunity for active learning. Many of the skills that students with histories of maltreatment need to learn (e.g., assertiveness, conflict resolution, initiating friendships) are best learned in a group format where there is opportunity for role-play and performance feedback.

5. In school settings, where children may be in groups with students they know or are getting to know but will see again, there is the possibility of establishing friendships. By connecting in a group, the beginnings of friendship may be established.

6. Groups are an efficient use of school-based clinicians' time. School practitioners' time can be used to serve multiple students simultaneously—an important feature, given time demands.

Bibliotherapy

Children and adolescents who have been maltreated may benefit from exposure to relevant literature. Books can be read in counseling sessions or at home, alone or with parents. Numerous resources exist, including books for children and adolescents who have been victims of various forms of maltreatment. For example, books regarding sexual abuse include *Feeling Good Again: A Workbook for Children 6 and Up Who Have Been Sexually Abused* (Wasserman, 1998), *It Happens to Boys Too* (Satullo & Bradway, 1987), and *How Long Does It Hurt?: A Guide to Recovering from Incest and Sexual Abuse for Teenagers, Their Friends, and Their Families* (Mather, Debye, & Wood, 1994). Similarly, books such as *When Mommy Got Hurt: A Story for Young Children about Domestic Violence* (Lee & Sylvester, 1997) or *A Family That Fights* (Bernstein, 1997) may be helpful to children exposed to domestic violence.

Model Programs

While the foregoing discussion about components, considerations, and resources may give school practitioners ideas for treatment planning, it may also be helpful to learn about model programs described in the literature. Certainly, Friedrich's integrated contextual model, described earlier in the chapter, is one very important example, but there are a number of others that may be useful to consider. School-based practitioners may replicate the program described or may use the model as a starting point to design their own modified version.

For example, one structured, time-limited therapy group for sexually abused preadolescent children has been described (Corder, Haizlip, & De-Boer, 1990). This treatment program incorporates a balance of affective, cognitive, and behavioral interventions. Cathartic exploration of feelings is prompted through art and storytelling exercises. Cognitive relabeling and self-esteem building are addressed through role-plays and games. Structured group exercises are designed to develop specific coping skills.

In another group model that has proved helpful for adolescent girls (Lindon & Nourse, 1994) three primary components are described: (1) a *skills component*, which allows clients to learn anxiety control (via relaxation and guided imagery), problem solving, assertiveness, and other social skills; (2) a *psychotherapeutic component* designed to facilitate the recognition of feelings, development of ego strength, identification with others, and peer relationships through the use of art, affective expression, and letter writing techniques; and (3) an *educative component* directly addressing sexuality and self-protection concerns. While large-scale program evaluations have not been reported, the program did report positive initial and 6-month follow-up results on a small sample (Lindon & Nourse, 1994).

Cohen and Mannarino (1993) have reported successfully on a short-term cognitive-behavioral treatment to address sexual abuse issues for young children and their caregivers. In the 12 treatment sessions, symptoms targeted included sexual behavior problems, aggression, sadness, and regressive behaviors.

Deblinger, McLeer, and Henry (1990) report on a pilot study on child abuse victims meeting the criteria for PTSD. This 12-session intervention includes gradual exposure aimed at disconnecting feelings of shame and anxiety from abuse-related stimuli, the modeling of positive coping behaviors, education, coping with anxiety, positive self-talk, and the expression of emotion. Parallel parenting groups focused on the parent's emotional responses, communication skills, and behavior management. Deblinger and Helfin (1996) have developed a related treatment manual which uses a cognitive-behavioral approach with sexually abused children and their nonoffending parents. While initial findings of all of these studies are promising, there is clearly the need for further empirical evaluation, particularly with controlled studies, comparing cognitive-behavioral approaches with others (Verduyn & Calam, 1999).

Kolko (1996b) describes and has evaluated another cognitive-behavioral program, but notes that the child component is based largely on a social learning premise. Kolko's program (1996b) is a child and parent program for physically abusive families. The children in this program, who are assumed to have had violent models, participate in sessions devoted to family stressors and violence, coping and self-control skills, training in interpersonal effectiveness, and instruction in skills use.

One very different but noteworthy model is Gil's play therapy for abused children (Gil, 1991). Play therapy assumes that the language of children is play, that, rather than sit in chairs and verbalize their "abuse issues" to work through them, children should use what comes naturally to them. The use of art or play media, rather than words, can provide an avenue for children to project their thoughts, feelings, and experiences.

In this model children are given some basic introductions, such as "I am someone who talks and plays with children. Sometimes I talk to kids about their thoughts and feelings. Other times, I play whatever the child wants" (Gil, 1991, p. 84). Some ground rules are also presented.

> "There are lots of things you can do in here. You can play with anything you see. You can talk if you want. You can play or draw. You choose what to do. Sometimes I might ask you questions. You can answer or not. There are a few rules. No hitting or breaking toys. No hurting yourself or me. All the toys stay here. . . . I'll set this timer and when the bell goes off, it's time to stop until the next time." (Gil, 1991, p. 85)

The child is then permitted to play with a variety of toys such as a sand tray with miniatures, a doll house with family dolls, nursing bottles, puppets, and art materials.

After these introductory activities, it is the therapist's role to observe the play, witnessing, reflecting, asking questions that help expand and explore, affectively and cognitively, themes that are generated. Children will frequently act out their abusive experiences in only slightly veiled ways. While, ideally, the play is a cathartic experience that allows the child to "work through" the traumatic material, there are times when the child becomes "stuck" and engages in "morbid play," in which he/she begins to retraumatize him/herself by repeating upsetting scenes over and over again. Should this occur, the therapist, using the play medium, interrupts this pattern and offers alternative solutions (e.g., another coping strategy, a rescuer, another way out, etc.) and helps the child to more successfully resolve the presented dilemma.

In addition to this "pure" model, play therapy approaches are frequently integrated with other theoretical approaches. For example, a therapist might use miniatures and a sand tray to allow the child to "role play" a conflict resolution approach. A child may be allowed to use art materials to create a picture of "the angry monster" inside and then be taught cognitive-behavioral ways to control the monster.

Additional Curricula

A number of curricula are available, which offer numerous treatment activity suggestions (including art, play, psychoeducational, and cognitive-behavioral approaches). Hindman's (1991) *When Mourning Breaks* is a particularly comprehensive example, with numerous exercises for varied ages. *Paper Dolls and Paper Airplanes: Therapeutic Exercises for Sexually Traumatized Children* (Crisci, Lay, & Lowenstein, 1998) is another nice example.

CONCLUSION

The treatment needs of children who have been maltreated are many and varied. School-based practitioners, with a solid grounding in the basics of trauma-focused work and drawing on model programs and available resources, are in a good position to promote recovery.

CHAPTER 6

Consulting with Teachers and Parents Regarding Child Maltreatment

♦

In many situations school psychologists, social workers, and counselors provide direct mental health services to children who have been abused. On other occasions, school professionals will make referrals to outside clinicians. Perhaps one of the most important roles for school mental health professionals, however, is consulting within the two systems most likely to have an influence on a child's life: the school and the home. Consulting with, informing, and supporting teachers and parents, the adults who likely have the most contact and influence on a child's life, may be among the most critical ways that school-based mental health professionals can truly make a difference in the lives of children who have been maltreated.

THE IMPORTANCE OF WORKING WITH TEACHERS

Vevier and Tharinger (1986) concluded that one of the key roles for school psychologists in responding to sexual abuse is the role of providing indirect services, that is, consulting with those who have "regular, ongoing contact with the child, that is, the 'front line' " (p. 306). Certainly this role is applicable to all forms of child maltreatment, as well. Teachers, administrators, and other school personnel may need assistance in responding. Teachers, in particular, must be supported in their "front line" roles. Given that they are with their students so many hours each day, teachers have the greatest opportunity to detect child abuse and the greatest opportunity for influence. Teachers, however, may be "frustrated with their own ineffectiveness in helping these troubled children to succeed in school." They "need support and encouragement for their persistent efforts" (Erickson & Egeland, 1987, p. 165).

Many of the child maltreatment-related topics and issues that teachers need assistance with can be addressed in multiple ways, including in-service training and formal and informal consultation. Teachers need basic information on child abuse and neglect, as it cannot be assumed that they received sufficient instruction in their college training. Additionally they need informed resources (Vevier & Tharinger, 1986) to keep them updated as the field's knowledge base grows and laws change. Teachers will also need assistance in applying the knowledge to situations with particular students.

Specific in-service training is important; through this means, many teachers can receive valuable information at the same time. School mental health professionals should advocate for at least annual opportunities to present this information to teachers. At the end of this chapter, outlines are presented that can be used to create handouts or overheads for this purpose. In addition to instruction regarding definitions, statistics, effects, and related topics, it may be helpful to show video clips of child abuse-related movies (e.g., *This Boy's Life, The Prince of Tides, Nuts*) or read excerpts of writings of child abuse survivors (e.g., Maya Angelou, David Pelzer). Through these media, teachers may gain a perspective that goes beyond intellectual understanding. Particularly for those teachers who have not experienced maltreatment in their own lives, seeing and hearing the stories may help them better appreciate the experience and perspectives of their students.

While in-service training is important, ongoing formal and informal consultation are also extremely valuable. A variety of consultation approaches may be helpful. For example, mental health consultation may have relevance in many cases. This perspective recognizes that, at times, the mental health issues of the consultee (e.g., a teacher) may interfere with objectivity (Caplan, 1995). Thus, rather than being given new information or told what to do, teachers often may benefit from the support of a mental health professional who assists them in recognizing their own feelings and addressing issues that may be interfering with their work with a particular child. This perspective may be particularly relevant when teachers are confronting the very emotionally laden issue of child maltreatment.

Given the high incidence and prevalence rates of child maltreatment, it should not be surprising to note that many teachers have histories of abuse or neglect in their own childhoods. These negative early life experiences may affect these adult survivor teachers' responses to their own students who may have been mistreated. Some may be hypersensitive. One teacher, for example, described herself as having a "savior complex," owing to her own history of abuse. Such teachers may become hypervigilant in their search for possible abuse cases or overly involved once they believe situations have been identified. Conversely, some teachers with a personal history of abuse may be dissociative or extraguarded because of the emotional distress caused by even considering that students in their class may be abused. One teacher, for example, acknowledged she probably "missed signals that abused kids in my classroom were giving me just because of my own abuse" (Tower, 1992, p. 12). These teachers, whether overly sensitive or overly avoidant, may need mental health consultation themselves or, in some cases, referrals for their own counseling so that they can work through their own concerns and be available to, but not overwhelmed by, their abused students.

Many teachers, fortunate enough to have been raised in supportive, healthy, nonabusive homes, may be somewhat naive and uninformed about the lives of children who suffer abuse. When they are first confronted with the unpleasant reality of many of their students' lives, the realization can be overwhelming. Once again, mental health consultation, including an opportunity for teachers to debrief them about their emotional experiences, may be valuable.

While mental health issues resulting in a lack of objectivity may be a factor that should be addressed in some consultation relationships, often this is not the only need. More commonly, teachers may be seeking consultation due to lack of knowledge, skills, and confidence. Thus, in addition to addressing any mental health concerns that do exist, consultants should be prepared to share content information regarding abuse and help the teacher plan a response to a particular child. Aspects of psychoeducational, problem solving, or behavioral consultation may be appropriate.

At times consultation, whether it be mental health-related or more content-based, may be done on a formal basis in which, for example, a teacher makes an appointment to discuss matters of concern with a school psychologist. More commonly, however, these discussions may be done on an informal basis as situations come up throughout the school day.

In either case, basic principles of good consultation, such as respecting teachers' expertise and problem solving together as partners, apply here. So, while teachers may be in need of content information, the process issues should still be respected. Thus, often a combination of mental health and problem-solving approaches may be helpful to both convey the needed information and suggestions and to address the potential obstacles to treatment adherence (Maital, 1996). Following is a discussion of a number of the topics or issues that, via in-service training or consultation, might be addressed with teachers.

Helping Teachers Identify Maltreatment

One of the most important aspects in supporting teachers is raising their awareness regarding the possibility that abuse could be happening—and likely *is* happening—in a few of their student's lives each year. Sharing incidence and prevalence rates may be a helpful reality check.

Additionally, helping teachers know what to look for may be critical. Teachers should be trained to notice general signs of internalized and externalized distress (e.g., anxiety, withdrawal, rageful aggression), which may or may not indicate abuse but are worthy of attention and evaluation to determine the cause. Additionally, they should be aware of more abuse-specific symptoms that more likely—though still not definitively—suggest abuse (e.g., a repeated pattern of a progression of bruises with inconsistent or suspicious explanations, sexual acting out). See Chapter 2 for a more detailed discussion of these matters.

Debunking such myths as "only poor kids are abused" or "I can tell by meeting a parent whether they could have done such a thing" may also serve a critical role. Teachers with these mistaken beliefs may overlook important clues to what may be going on in students' lives (even in the lives of middle-class students with "nice" parents).

Additionally, it is important to impress on teachers (especially elementary teachers) that they have the unique opportunity to spend several hours with a child away from his/her home (where most abuse occurs). Few, if any, other concerned adults will have similar access to the child. Teachers should be encouraged to avoid a "diffusion of responsibility," wherein everyone assumes *someone else* has done something, will do something, or should do something. Many children who were abused for years likely demonstrated signs that were ignored or exhibited symptoms that were not detected.

Teachers do not need to become paranoid or overly focused on looking for signs of abuse. Clearly, those in supportive, consultative roles must understand that teachers are educators, not social workers. At the same time, teachers should be encouraged to take advantage of naturally occurring opportunities. An essay in an English class spontaneously written about an abusive household should be followed by statements or questions that invite the possibility of further dialogue, such as "I was struck by how sad that girl was in your story" (and see if the student chooses to identify and disclose) or "Where did get your ideas?" Teachers can casually inquire about injuries or distress that children talk about or are evident. "Wow, Charlie, how did you get that black eye?" "You've been complaining about your back hurting for some time—what happened?" "I appreciate your after-school help with the bulletin boards, but you said you don't want to go home. What's going on?"

Teachers should also know what to do if a child, in a follow-up to these questions or spontaneously, discloses abuse. Ideally, the teacher can follow the steps discussed in Chapter 2 regarding handling disclosures. Since the child obviously feels comfortable with the teacher, if a teacher is able, it is preferable for her to calmly manage the conversation herself rather than asking the child to "Stop! Go tell the school psychologist." Passing the student on to someone else may seem confusing to the child. The child may not want to disclose the information to a school mental health professional (who may be a stranger to the child). Such a move may inadvertently send unintended messages to a child that "this is more than I can handle—you are on your own" or "I don't want to talk to you now that you've told me this—something is wrong with you." If the teacher is not comfortable handling the conversation, other options can be considered and should be handled as sensitively as possible. For example, as the child begins to tell her story, the teacher might say, "Wow, Mary. This sounds very important. There is someone at school that can help us. Do you remember our social worker, Ms. Ramirez. I think she'll have some ideas about what we can do. I'll go with you and you can tell us both what happened."

It is preferable to not have the child repeat the story too many times at school (e.g., first with the teacher, then the principal, then the social worker) because there will likely be even more interviews by child protective services and/or police and/or attorneys. Multiple interviews may be distressing to the child and may contribute to concerns regarding the accuracy of the child's testimony, especially since concerns about "leading questions" increase with each interview. Also, the child may begin to think that adults must be looking for different answers simply because "they keep asking."

In sum, teachers should be informed, aware, and willing to follow up on possible signs or disclosures of abuse. Teachers may need information, consultation, and support in these roles.

Assistance with Reporting Dilemmas

Another critical area in which teachers may need consultation and support is in handling reporting dilemmas. Recall from Chapter 3 that teachers, while frequent reporters of child abuse, are also likely the greatest underreporters (O'Toole et al., 1999). A recent survey of educators found that few felt they really understood the reporting laws and many were eager to have additional in-service training (Crenshaw et al., 1995).

In-service instruction covering basic information regarding the law, teacher's mandated reporter status, the phone numbers to reach child protective services, and the written report requirements should be offered fairly frequently. Certainly they should be included in all new teacher training sessions. Signs or posters in the teachers' lounge and flyers in mail boxes may be important reminders for all.

However, teachers need more than these basics. In-service and consultation formats should allow teachers to address their concerns and hesitancies about reporting. Frequently when teachers do not report, it is not because they are not aware of the law, do not understand that they are mandated reporters, or do not have the correct phone numbers. While the lack of such basic information, in some instances, is a problem, there are typically other issues involved in decisions not to report. Fears, personal concerns, lack of administrative support, and frustrations with the child protection system are often interfering and must be addressed directly. Teachers may need opportunities to vent their frustrations and to be included in problem-solving efforts to ensure that these obstacles do not interfere with reports being made and children being protected.

After the Abuse Report

Teachers' involvement goes beyond identifying and reporting abuse. Teachers who make an abuse report or who, for some other reason, are aware that students in their class may have been victims of child abuse need ongoing support.

Interacting with the Family

Teachers may need support in their "after-the-abuse-report" dealings with the family. Frequently there are fears that the family will retaliate. Fortunately, most of the time these fears are not realized (Tower, 1992). Child abuse offenders are not typically a threat to adults outside of their family. Certainly, if threats have been made, however, teachers should be supported in getting whatever security support fits the situation, including police involvement as appropriate. In most cases, teachers should not assume that parents who may have abused or neglected their children do not care about their children or are "all bad." Rarely are situations so black and white. Families who have abused their children vary dramatically but not uncommonly include some combination of the following parental variables: drug and/or alcohol addictions, immaturity, unresolved histories of abuse and neglect, financial stressors, poor coping skills, and limited social skills.

In spite of their poor choices and negative situations, most parents do have some genuine concern for their children and should be treated with that assumption by those at school. Teachers are wise to allow CPS or law enforcement to take whatever more confrontive or adversarial position may be necessary.

Additionally, teachers may need help in understanding the role of the nonoffending parent (if any). Teachers may tend to be upset with the "sick" mother, for example, who "must have known" that her child was being sexually abused by her husband. Teachers may need to be reminded that mothers of children who have been sexually abused represent a heterogeneous group. Far from being the center of the pathological system, as 1960s professional literature tended to characterize her, many mothers of sexually abused children are mentally healthy, honestly did not know about the abuse, and acted supportively once it was disclosed (Tharinger, 1991; Tharinger & Horton, 1992). While certainly there are cases in which the mother consciously chose not to see the abuse or even colluded in it, teachers should not assume that this was the case. In the majority of cases, it was not.

Similarly, teachers and other school personnel may be frustrated with mothers in domestic violence situations. Teachers may have stereotypes of women in domestic violence situations who "are so dependent on a man" that they will "subject their children" to witnessing the violence rather than "have the guts" to leave him. It is important for teachers to understand that, typically, domestic violence situations are much more complicated than this. For example, it may be helpful for a teacher to fully realize that, if a woman is genuinely fearful of her violent partner, she may be accurate in assuming that her life and the lives of her children are most in danger when she leaves him (Edleson, 1999a). Additionally, if a battered woman does manage to leave safely, the odds are that there will be court-ordered child visitation and she may be forced to have her children visit their violent father without her to protect them. Worse, he may successfully sue for sole custody. Studies have demonstrated that batterers are more likely than other fathers to sue for, and gain, custody of their children (Stahley & Adamson, 1990). Thus, the dilemmas of a battered woman are complicated. Often what appears to be choices that are callous to her children's needs are in fact difficult choices made in an effort to protect her children (Edleson, 1999a). While, ideally, the social service, law enforcement, and judicial systems will work in such a way that the mother and children can be kept safe and the perpetrator of the violence can be held accountable, situations do not always work out that way. Even in the best of circumstances, it frequently takes time to successfully resolve matters.

In sum, in either of these, or any other, child maltreatment situations, teachers are advised to not be quick to make negative assumptions about nonoffending mothers (or nonoffending fathers). The nonoffending parent's ability to stay mentally healthy (e.g., not depressed), psychologically available, and engaged in a positive relationship with her (or his) child will be critically predictive of the child's trauma outcome (Tharinger, 1991; Tharinger & Horton, 1992). Thus, first of all, teachers and all school personnel should be reminded that, in many cases, the stereotypical assumptions simply are not accurate. Second, regardless of the choices the mother (in the great majority of cases) has made up to this point, it is in the best interest of the child for school personnel to encourage and support her. If teachers give direct or indirect messages of disdain or distrust of the parent, this may contribute to overwhelming stress, depression, and inability to provide the support that her child needs. To the degree that a parent is supported, encouraged, and able to be available, her children will benefit.

Responding to the Children

In addition to responding to the families, teachers must decide how they will respond to the students who have been abused. Long after reports have been made and child protective decisions have been determined (regardless of the outcome), teachers will have abused children in their classrooms. While certainly all children benefit from a competent, caring teacher, those with an abuse history may have a greater need to have a special attachment with a concerned teacher (Gelardo & Sanford, 1987). This relationship may be particularly powerful among younger elementary school students who typically spend the majority of the school day with one special teacher (Erickson & Egeland, 1987).

Teachers, by providing a positive, consistent presence, can assist in giving children who have been abused some of what they have missed. Many researchers and writers in the abuse field have pointed out, in various ways, that children who are abused not only suffer from the acts of commission (e.g., physical assault, sexual fondling, etc.) but also typically from acts of omission. Put simply, it is not only what abused children "get"—it is equally what they "*don't* get." For example, Margolin (1998) has discussed that, ideally, parents are actively engaged in multiple roles for their children, including the following: providers of emotional support, models of emotional regulation, facilitators of relationships outside the family, and disciplinarians. Margolin points out that many of these parenting roles are compromised when there is domestic violence, and the same is true in many forms of abuse, as well.

Thus, one of the important goals for teachers may be to try to, in some small ways, fill these voids. For example, if the teacher can provide these students with some extra emotional support via extra encouragement, a few minutes of time before or after class to listen, or assisting the child in joining groups of children that are likely to be a positive influence, it would be most helpful. Teachers who directly teach social skills such as anger management, emotional expression, and conflict resolution (or invite school psychologists or social workers into their classrooms to do so) may provide a valuable service to children who did not have an opportunity to learn these skills at home. Teachers who demonstrate healthy emotional regulation act as important role models. Those who provide a positive connection, then, are making a meaningful difference in a number of arenas.

Unfortunately, there are a number of dynamics that may interfere with this ideally positive relationship, of which the two most significant ones may be teachers' stereotypes and students' behaviors.

One potential obstacle to a healthy response by teachers is stereotyping or stigmatization that may inadvertently occur. While, in general, it would seem like a good idea to keep teachers informed and updated regarding child abuse issues and common effects, there is the potential iatrogenic effect that should be mentioned. Teachers may, in some cases, begin to feel sorry for, and/or expect less of children whom they know, or suspect, have been abused. This, certainly, would not work to the children's advantage.

Browne and Finkelhor, in 1986, first raised the concern about the possibility of stigmatization of the abused child, particularly in cases of sexual abuse. Empirical research regarding teachers' attitudes has been mixed. In one noteworthy study, teachers expected less future success in students who had been sexually abused (Bromfield, Bromfield, & Weiss, 1988). A more recent investigation, however, resulted in more hopeful findings. In this study, teachers did not have globally negative views about sexually abused children. They only specifically expected that these students would be under more stress. Such an assumption is fairly accurate and is not indicative of stigmatization (O'Donohue & O'Hare, 1997). While the more recent research is promising, those consulting, supporting, and training teachers want to keep this potential phenomenon of stigmatization in mind as something to be avoided.

Unfortunately, this is not the only challenge to a positive student–teacher relationship. Although there is a growing awareness and sensitivity to the problem of child maltreatment, given the multiple symptom patterns described in earlier chapters, it is understandable that many teachers find it difficult to act upon their concerns. Many children who have been abused or neglected will internalize their distress, act fearful, withdraw, and avoid connections. This pattern may make it difficult for teachers to develop any type of special relationship. Other children who have been abused may externalize their distress, acting aggressively, defiantly, or even exhibiting sexual behavior problems. These symptoms, which certainly can be emotionally upsetting to the teacher and disruptive to the classroom structure and routine (Milgram, 1984), may make it difficult for a teacher to even like, much less develop a special connection with, those particular students. Without support from the school's professionals, teachers may be drawn into a classroom replication of the child's destructive family relationships (Erickson & Egeland, 1987).

While challenging, these two potential obstacles—teachers' stereotypes and students' symptoms—are not insurmountable; however, they are not insignificant. Teachers need support and encouragement for their persistent efforts to be patient and understanding of children who have been maltreated. The discussion of these obstacles illustrates the need for information to be provided to teachers, not simply a list of "indicators" and "effects" of abuse in children. Teachers need support and information to know how to address the ongoing needs of these students.

Theoretical Understanding

Sometimes it may be helpful for a teacher to have some conceptual understanding of why children who have been abused may act as they do. The following theoretical explanations may be shared in an in-service training session or consultation. School psychologists or other mental health professionals may use these theories to assist by helping to reinterpret a child's behavior to a teacher, thus helping the teacher to avoid a classroom replication of the child's destructive family relationships (Erickson & Egeland, 1987).

Social learning theory (Bandura, 1977) would suggest that children who have seen violence—particularly violence at the hands of those closest to them—have learned to be violent. While a teacher may teach other skills, it will take some time to "unlearn" what has been modeled to the child. In many cases there may be continued models of violence in their home, in their neighborhoods, and on TV. Thus, one lesson of "stop and think" taught at school has a hard time competing with multiple models of "when you're mad, you can be violent."

> Juan, a second grader, was regularly beaten physically by his stepfather, Mr. Estrada. Juan also witnessed Mr. Estrada abuse the others in his home. Ms. Steinway, his teacher, knew things had been bad in Juan's family but did not know the details. What was evident in the classroom, however, was that Juan "had a temper." Whenever Juan had a conflict with other children, he would explode into violence, punching, hitting, or yelling at his peers. Juan had learned to be violent by watching his stepfather. While Ms. Steinway, together with the school psychologist, had taught some basic anger management lessons to the class, they did not seem effective with Juan. His stepfather had, for years, taught Juan a different lesson.

> Although Ms. Steinway should be encouraged to continue to teach the anger management and other social skills to her class, she may also need support to understand that these lessons may take a while to "sink in" with Juan. Additionally, the teacher should recognize that among the most powerful ways of influencing him is through her positive modeling of prosocial skills (Lorber, Felton, & Reid, 1985).

Social information-processing models (Crick & Dodge, 1996) would suggest that a child who has been abused has "made sense" of what he/she has experienced. A hostile attribution bias (a view that the world is out to get him/her) and a perspective that retaliation is legitimate and should be immune from consequences is understandable, given the life experiences of abused students (Dodge et al., 1995; O'Donohue & Rudman, 1999).

> Mr. Tyler was surprised by Sean's aggressive response when someone accidentally spilled food on him in the cafeteria. Sean seemed to have a habit of overreacting like this that Mr. Tyler could not understand. He did not real-

ize that Sean, who had a horrific history of abuse, had learned to believe others were "out to get him." Sean rarely considered the possibility that a spill in the cafeteria would be an accident. Instead, he jumped to the conclusion that peers would do such things just to bother him and that they were "picking on him." Given his history of abuse, this perception is understandable, though not accurate. Part of Mr. Tyler's role in assisting Sean was to try to "chip away" at these negative assumptions by gently challenging the thinking, pointing out contradictory evidence, and offering other possible explanations.

The *PTSD perspective* (Famularo, Fenton, Kincherff, Ayoub, & Barnum, 1994; Wolfe, Sas, & Wekerle, 1994) explains that, much like a veteran of war, a child who is abused has been exposed to too much, too soon, to the point of being psychologically overwhelmed. Just as a veteran may struggle with flashbacks or jump to the sound of a car backfiring, a child who has been abused (experienced a war of sorts in his/her own household) may exhibit what appears to be, to those who do not understand, bizarre behavior. Symptoms include a recurrent reexperiencing of the stressor, avoidance of reminders of the abuse, and persistent hyperarousal, including a sense of "hypervigilance" (i.e., always being on guard against "potentially dangerous" people or situations) (House, 1999).

> Sally's behavior puzzled Ms. Moyer. Knowing that Sally had a difficult past (the adoptive parents had been quite open), Ms. Moyer tried to be patient and encouraging. When Sally seemed to "space out" for extended periods in class, Ms. Moyer tried to reach out to be encouraging to Sally with a pat on the back or other form of physical connection. Sally, rather than seeming to appreciate these gestures, pulled back or flinched. Initially Ms. Moyer was somewhat hurt. "What is her problem? I'm just trying to be nice." With some consultation, Ms. Moyer could appreciate that Sally's experience with touch had not been positive, but rather sexually or physically abusive. Thus, her touch "triggered" bad memories and made Sally fear what might happen next. Ms. Moyer quickly understood Sally's behavior and realized that creating a safe atmosphere in the classroom may positively influence Sally.

Attachment theory (Alexander, 1992; Karen, 1994) suggests that if a child, for example, in a multiproblem, chaotic, abusive household is not able to securely attach to a primary caregiver, the internal working model is compromised. That is, the child does not have an opportunity to develop a positive view about him/herself ("I am worth love") or the world ("people are there when I need them"). The child who does not have the opportunity to develop a secure attachment may have difficulty in forming stable relationships with others, and, again, the patient teacher must gently challenge the working model by being safe, consistent, and reasonably available. Some students, particularly young children, may regard the teacher as their first safe caregiver.

Joe was an angry student. Coach Taylor had certainly noticed Joe's constant verbal assaults on team members. He seemed to be constantly posturing to be the "tough guy" of the seventh grade. Coach also noticed that Joe was most harsh on himself. Once, after a game, Coach found Joe in the locker room kicking the locker and yelling at himself, "You're stupid, stupid, stupid! You lost the game. It was your stupid move." Coach Taylor tried to encourage Joe that he had done his best and to ask him what else was going on, but to no avail. Joe just ran away. Coach Taylor remained a steady, encouraging influence, whether or not Joe seemed to appreciate it. Little by little, though, Joe started spending more time with Coach Taylor, opening up just a little, seeming to enjoy the positive connection. After he graduated from high school, Joe came back to thank his coach. Joe explained that his life had been full of abuse. Joe's father, a violent alcoholic, had been a frightening figure in his life, and his mother, who had collapsed into permanent depression, was also unavailable to him. Joe had grown up with no safe base, hating himself, believing the lies his father would yell in a drunken rage. Joe had been afraid to let anybody help him. He just wanted Coach Taylor to know what a difference he had made by being a steady positive influence.

Sometimes, teachers may be frustrated with the degree of passivity, "lack of motivation," and attitudes of helplessness that they see in some children who have been maltreated. If teachers can consider that many of these children may have been in truly helpless situations, the dilemma and the solutions may be clearer.

The *learned helplessness paradigm* (Seligman, 1975) has been applied to the understanding of abuse victims. Consider the original classic experiment. Dogs were shocked on one side of the cage and would move to the other side until a fence prevented them from reaching the other "shock-free" side. For a time, when shocked, the dogs would frantically try to reach the other side, but they eventually learned that their efforts were futile. Ultimately, the dogs would not even attempt to move to the other side, having learned that there was no use. The dogs simply lay down and endured the shocks. Later, the fence was removed. The dogs were shocked and free to move elsewhere, but they still just lay down and endured the shocks. They had learned to be helpless. The dogs had learned it was "no use" trying. Trainers had to engage in repeated trials of pulling the dogs over the line (where the fence had been) to retrain the dogs that moving was again a true painless option: the fence was no longer there; they could control their outcomes; they did not have to be shocked.

Now consider children who have been abused. They have been in horrible, "shocking" situations. There was a "fence" that prevented them from getting relief. Many times, the very adults that should have been protecting and nurturing them were the ones who were "shocking them." Thus, as dependents, their efforts at escape would have been futile. They could not "get over the fence." They learned to "lie down" and take it, too, and at some level to recognize their helplessness. The problem is that they have generalized the experience. Now, even when there is no fence, they still lie down, so to speak. Briere (1992) explains the phenomenon succinctly: "Not only may child victims come to accept the extent to which avoidance of abuse is beyond their control, they may subsequently generalize this assumption to other, less uncontrollable, events, and respond accordingly" (p. 26). Teachers, then, must at some level consider themselves trainers to "pull children over the line," to help them repeatedly experience the reality that "you can get away from the shocks."

Susie had been sexually abused by her stepfather and older stepbrothers. Since they had threatened her life and her mother's life (and she had reason to believe them, given the domestic violence that she had witnessed) if she told anyone, she kept quiet for 3 years. She was helpless. When finally her mother did find out by walking in on an incident, her mother took immediate action. She immediately moved away with Susie to another state and reported the incident to CPS. Susie and her mother were safe. As Susie started at a new junior high school, however, teachers began noticing some alarming patterns. They found that Susie was allowing other students to cheat by copying from her tests or letting them use her homework. Initially teachers interpreted this behavior as that of a new student desperate to make friends. After all, she certainly seemed very sad and lonely. Then, one day, a hall monitor observed a disturbing scene: Susie was being teased mercilessly, poked, prodded by her peers—and she seemed to "just take it." Susie had never reported this type of behavior to any teachers or administrators. As a matter of fact, Susie rarely spoke to any teachers or administrators about anything.

Susie had been in a helpless situation with her stepfather for several years. In her mind, to stay alive and keep her mother alive, she had had to "endure the shocks" of abuse. She had learned that "the fence was up" and there was no point in trying. Even though she had now moved to a safe situation, and thus "the fence had been removed," her learned pattern was still continuing. It may not actually occur to Susie that she has any other option than simply to "put up with" kids cheating, teasing, or degrading her. Options such as sticking up for herself, asking for help from teachers, or letting her mother know what is going on may not even occur to her. Teachers may have initially viewed Susie as trying to "buy friends," but with a better understanding of learned helplessness they can see that she is acting the way she has been taught to act. The school's job then, at least in part, is to encourage Susie in ways that teach her that she can in many situations influence, if not completely control, her circumstances. Some things are shocking, but there is often no fence.

The above discussions demonstrate just a sampling of the range of theories that have been suggested to explain the effects of maltreatment on the victim, his/her feelings, thoughts, and behavior. Any of a variety of theoretical approaches may be selected to help a teacher understand the disturbing internalizing and externalizing behaviors of children who have been abused. In an in-service training format it may be helpful to present a number of these ideas. In a consultation regarding a particular child, the mental health profession may choose the "best fit" for a particular situation.

APPLICATIONS FOR TEACHERS

While each theory offers a unique perspective, there are some important classroom implications that cut across theoretical orientations.

1. *Providing opportunities for success and teaching tangible skills (academic, artistic, or athletic) are valuable roles for teachers.* Teachers who can provide a "rich schedule of reinforcement" (Stark, Rouse, & Livingston, 1991), many compliments, words of encouragement, shaping comments, etc., will contribute positively to the life of a maltreated child. There is some evidence (Kolko, 1996a) that, in the case of children who have been physically abused, it is the lack of positive reinforcement from their parents (rather than the physical abuse itself) that is most damaging.

Children who have been maltreated have typically had numerous experiences that have contributed to a negative view of themselves (e.g., "the damaged goods syndrome," common among those who have been sexually abused). It may be helpful, naturally, for them to have a more tangibly positive way to think of themselves. Instead of "I'm the dirty one that Dad did those nasty things to," a child can begin to think, "I am the smart one who is good at math," "the fast one who is good at sports," or "the artistic one who is talented at sketching portraits." One social worker who worked with quite troubled abused youth taught origami as a means to help the children feel positive about themselves and have a unique talent.

2. *Patience is a necessity; change takes time.* Even after the abuse has stopped, inappropriate behaviors do not typically end immediately. In fact, often the problematic behaviors get worse before they get better. Teachers must understand that immediate drastic change is often not possible—for a number of reasons. First, teachers must understand they are "chipping away" at entrenched patterns of thinking and behaving that may have been familiar to the child and the family for years. Additionally, it is important to recognize that symptoms once served a useful purpose (e.g., "spacing out," when emotional or sexual abuse was going on; running away or lying, if a mistake was made, to avoid physical abuse) (Erickson & Egeland, 1987), so they are not easily dropped. Finally, teachers should be reminded that the external factors in a child's life frequently become more stressful after a disclosure. Any num-

ber of the following stressors might occur in a child's life *after* the abuse has been disclosed or discovered: the child might be punished or ridiculed, or called a liar for making the report; the parents may experience elevated levels of conflict or violence in their relationship; there may be multiple interviews and court appearances; parents may separate; one or both parents may be incarcerated; the family income level may drop considerably after the disappearance, removal, or incarceration of one parent; the family may decide to move; the family may endure major financial stressors. Thus, while school personnel might be thinking, "Why isn't this kid getting better? I thought we reported the abuse, so things would be better for him," the reality may be that, at least initially, the child is enduring more stressful life events than ever (Tharinger, 1991).

3. *The classroom must be a safe environment.* Children who have been abused need teachers to exercise enough control to keep things from feeling chaotic, unpredictable, and unsafe. Nonviolence and positive conflict resolution should certainly be directly taught, and violence of any kind (physical, verbal, threats, etc.) must not be allowed. Sexual abuse or harassment of fellow students, at any level, cannot be tolerated.

Children who have been abused may be more prone than their peers to be the victims or the perpetrators of school teasing, bullying, or other violence. Teachers must help children to avoid falling into either of these roles.

4. *Teachers should avoid stereotypes, remembering that not all abused children are alike.* Children who have been abused represent a wide range of types, personality characteristics, and emotional needs (Horton & Cruise, 1997b). Abuse experiences vary dramatically. One student may have been fondled once by a camp director, while another may have been sexually abused, including being subjected to intercourse for years by her father. One child may have endured three weeks of being slapped around by the mother's new boyfriend, while another may have been subjected to life-threatening violence by both parents his/her entire life. Factors such as frequency, duration, and severity of the abuse may vary considerably, but even those factors do not entirely predict a child's outcome. A child's personal characteristics (IQ, temperament, etc.), cognitions about the abuse and life in general, disclosure experiences, and the degree of others' support in the aftermath will also vary significantly, resulting in an infinite variety of possible responses to the trauma. Children who have been abused—just as with children who have not—must be treated as the individuals that they are; stereotypes are not fair to anyone. Their personal unique development should be supported strenuously and vigorously.

5. *Behaviors still need to be addressed.* When consulting with teachers regarding children who have been maltreated, it is certainly important to help instill a compassionate, understanding approach by providing some theoretical understanding and some of the practical suggestions discussed above. At

the same time, it should be clear that being compassionate does not mean not addressing the problematic behaviors. It does not do a child a favor for the teacher to assume the attitude that the child "cannot help it" because of the abuse. Teachers, in addressing either internalized or externalized behavior problems, must balance compassion with expectations for change.

Internalized Distress

A child who is withdrawn and refuses to join in any social activities at school or a student who "just doesn't feel up to" doing any homework needs the teacher to gently encourage progress. Certainly children who are introverted should have their needs for solitude respected (Horton & Oakland, 1996). Time for working and playing alone should be available. It is a different matter, however, if a student is avoiding interactions with classmates owing to a deep-seated depression or anxiety that is perhaps the result of abuse. In that case, contact with peers and productive activity will be important to encourage.

Depression

Teachers must understand that, when children (or adults for that matter) are depressed, they often "don't feel like" doing what would be good for them to do (Stark et al., 1991). This can result in a downward spiral. Imagine, as an example, a third-grade student, Hannah, who has had a difficult life and has learned not to expect much in the future. Years of abuse have left her depressed and hopeless. Hannah does not feel inclined to invite friends to do something with her, and she does not feel like joining their activities either; she is just too sad. This minimal social interaction is common among depressed children but inhibits positive social contacts (Stark et al., 1991). Given her habit of withdrawal, Hannah has not developed friendships, so she feels more lonely, isolated, and sad. These feelings cause her to withdraw even more, and the vicious cycle continues. To add to the downward spiral, peers often interpret depressed peers' behaviors negatively, in a way that decreases the likelihood that they will continue to invite interaction ("She doesn't look like she wants to play with us, so we won't invite her." "Hannah is looking away from us. Doesn't she like us anymore?" etc.). Hannah interprets her peers' lack of invitations as a sign of rejection, and another round of the cycle continues.

Teachers may have opportunities to gently challenge the pattern and get the cycle going in a more positive direction. By making "study buddy" arrangements or pairing children for games at recess (carefully choosing the right partner, of course), the teacher may help a depressed child to engage in some positive peer interactions.

Anxiety

Children who have been maltreated have grown up in situations that were less than safe, stable, or affirming. Thus, it is not surprising that many abused children have heightened levels of anxiety, a phenomenon important for teachers to understand. Put simply, avoidance is the natural tendency of an anxious individual. A student who is anxious about giving a speech might well miss class on the day he/she was to make a presentation. Avoidance, unfortunately, just fuels the anxiety. Postponing the speech only made the student more nervous. Similarly, a young child may avoid joining in a game due to anxious feelings; however, avoiding the contact makes it worse. For the moment, the child's choice has been negatively reinforced (no social contact, no discomfort; the aversive has been avoided) (House, 1999), but ultimately, nothing is solved. The idea of joining the next day becomes even more difficult. It is this pattern that can keep adults confined to their homes or "unable" to have social contacts. Typically, what can be helpful is successive gradual exposure to more and more challenging situations (Kendall et al., 1991), allowing for successes along the way. To force a highly anxious child into the leading role of a school play to "help her get over it," for example, is likely to backfire, adding another negative experience and increasing the odds of further anxiety and avoidance. Instead, helping a child experience mildly anxiety-producing situations successfully and moving up gradually to more challenging situations is better. Encouraging attendance at a school play with a chosen partner may be the best "first step." With this successful experience under his/her belt, the student may be prepared to become more involved the next year.

Externalizing Behaviors

Just as teachers should challenge children to move beyond their internalizing symptoms, externalizing symptoms, too, should not be considered permanent. "Poor Chadman. He can't help himself. I know that his family was very violent. He's just doing the same thing." Clearly, adopting this attitude would not promote safety for the other children in the classroom, but equally importantly this would not help Chadman in his development. Being allowed to bully, regardless of abuse background, will only cause more problems. Negative relationships with peers would likely develop, the patterns would become entrenched, and the likelihood of continued violence, criminality, and substance abuse would increase. The compassionate response to Chadman, in fact, is to understand the possible source of the problem behaviors *and* help him begin to change them as soon as possible. By expecting him to change these behaviors, the teacher gives Chadman the hope of a more positive future.

In responding to children who have aggressive and other externalizing behavior problems, teachers should receive consultation regarding general best-practice strategies for these issues. Teachers frequently feel "deskilled" in addressing the needs of abused children and may need to be reminded to do what they would do with any other children demonstrating such problematic behaviors. The use of standard practices such as setting clear rules, expectations, and consequences should be encouraged, as long as these are delivered in a positive, affirming way that does not re-create harsh, ridiculing experiences from abusive homes. Discussing with the child the natural consequences of behavior choices ("I see the other kids avoid you after you explode like that; I'm afraid you won't have many friends if this continues") may be important. Offering social problem solving and cognitive and behavioral alternatives may also be helpful (Lochman, White, & Wayland, 1991). "Charlie, I think maybe Darren knocked your tower down on accident" or "I know it is hard for you when you get so angry you just want to throw things down or hurt someone. We don't allow that in the class, but if you can tell me you need a break, we can have a plan where you can step outside the classroom for a moment and calm down." Prompts to use skills the child is learning in the classroom or in group or individual counseling may be valuable. "Erin, I see you getting kind of frustrated. Would this be a time to take a few deep breaths and relax a bit before working on this math worksheet some more?" In some cases a nonverbal signal may be worked out as a prompt that is just between the teacher and the student.

In addition to addressing general externalizing behavior problems, teachers may need specialized support and consultation in handling a particular type of acting out, namely, sexual behavior problems. At times, teachers may be confronted by unusual sexual behavior by children they know have been abused, while at other times it may be children's inappropriate sexual behavior at school that provides necessary clues to detect sexual abuse.

A key aspect of providing help is assisting school personnel in distinguishing between normal and problematic sexual behavior among children (Horton, 1996). The related literature (e.g., Berliner & Rawlings, 1991; Gil & Johnson, 1993) describes a number of factors to consider in making such determinations. Those consulting with teachers who have concerns about students' sexual behaviors can assist by helping teachers think through the following questions.

1. *Are there any power differences between the children involved?* Examples of potential power differences include differences in age, size, strength, social status, or intellectual ability. When there is sexual behavior between children of unequal power, there is more cause for concern. For example, if a teacher discovers two kindergarten students playing some version of "you show me yours, I'll show you mine," the level of concern and reaction to this situation

should be markedly different than were the same scenario to occur between a sixth grader and a kindergartner.

2. *What was the affect of the children involved when "caught" by school personnel?* If two third-grade boys were involved in fairly innocent, curious sexual play or discussion in the rest room, some giggly embarrassment may be the reaction to school personnel walking in. However, if the children's reactions are more intense, such as extreme shame, anger, or anxiety, this may suggest something more serious may be involved.

3. *What was the student's response to correction or redirection?* A child who immediately responds to a teacher's instructions should cause less concern than a child who compulsively and/or defiantly repeats the sexual behavior in spite of a teacher's directions. For example, it may not be unusual for young children to engage in some masturbation, even in public situations such as the classroom. However, in most cases, a simple clear direction from the teacher (such as "Johnny, we don't touch our private parts at school; let's keep hands on the desk") will settle the matter once and for all. Children who seem to ignore these directions, either because of an apparent compulsion or an intentional effort to upset the teacher, are displaying more serious behaviors.

4. *What specific sexual behaviors were involved?* While "show-me-yours-and-I'll-show-you-mine" type behaviors, or doctor games, are not appropriate in the school setting, they are most likely indicative of normal sexual curiosity and not nearly as deserving of concern as actions involving attempted intercourse or other imitation of adult sexual behaviors.

5. *What means did the child who initiated the sexual activity use to gain compliance from the others involved?* School personnel should be most concerned when force, threats of force, or coercive techniques (such as bribes or social threats) are used.

6. *How does the sexual behavior fit into the whole of a child's life?* A student who engages in some sexual talk or behavior but has numerous other academic, athletic, and social interests likely is involved in qualitatively different situation than a child for whom sexual behavior and concerns are interfering with or replacing appropriate activities or interests for that particular developmental level (Berliner & Rawlings, 1991; Gil & Johnson, 1993).

Teachers and other school personnel should understand that children's sexual development is just as much a part of normal growth as social, cognitive, or physical development. Sexual discussion or behavior that is time-limited, involves children of similar ages, and appears to be indicative of curiosity in understanding one's own and others' bodies is generally no great cause for alarm (Johnson, 1990). While school personnel may want to inform parents that a child engages in these behaviors at school so that parents can be aware and enforce school personnel's instructions to the child, there is likely no need for further action. For example, a teacher might have a discussion such as the following with a parent, "Mrs. Darman, just so you know, Holly was talking a lot about childbirth today, and tried to pull down her pants to show the others exactly where babies 'come out.' I suspect, with the new addition to your family, there have been related conversations at home. I simply told her we would let the other children's parents explain these things to the other kids and that we all needed to keep our clothes on at school."

If, on the other hand, the answers to the questions above lead school personnel to conclude that the behaviors are beyond normal, the reaction should be different. If the child engaging in these inappropriate behaviors was not known to have been sexually abused, depending on the severity of the situation and the parents' response, a report should be considered. If the child has already been identified as a child who has been sexually abused the teacher should keep parents informed of the ongoing concerns, and, with appropriate parental permissions (see Chapter 4), the child's therapist should be apprised.

In either case, teachers may need very specific suggestions and guidelines regarding supervision and appropriate interventions (Slater & Gallagher, 1989). Children with severe sexual acting out may be placed in a more restrictive environment (e.g., self-contained special education classes, alternative schools, or residential placements for sexually aggressive children). Children whose behavior would be classified at the less severe end of the continuum may be appropriately supervised and supported in the regular classroom. School psychologists, social workers, administrators, teachers, and others on decision-making teams must balance the goal of maintaining the least restrictive environment for the child against the need to protect other children who could become future victims. Factors that should be carefully considered include the nature of the child's sexual behavior; the number of known incidents; the power difference between the perpetrating child and the victim(s); the response to being caught; comorbidity with other aggressive/impulsive problems; parental reactions; and the level of supervision reasonably available in various settings.

Supervision Plans

Assisting teachers in determining supervision plans for children with sexual behavior problems may be a difficult challenge. Supporting the child's full recovery is an important goal. Teachers should be encouraged not to, in any way, stigmatize the child or be overly pessimistic about his/her ability to change the behavioral pattern. In most cases, these children are victims of abuse, are reenacting what they have been exposed to, and should be viewed "compassionately and hopefully" (Friedrich, 1993). At the same time, school personnel, for both ethical and legal liability reasons, must also be concerned about protecting other children. Supervision is central to meeting both of these objectives. Without close supervision, a child who acts out sexually cannot be successfully maintained in, or transitioned back to, a regular school setting.

Teachers may appreciate assistance in developing a specific plan of supervision. Individual plans will vary, depending on the specific needs of the child and the class setting. In general, however, *children who have demonstrated significant sexual behavior problems should not be left unsupervised with any other child for any amount of time.* In most school settings, particularly in elementary schools, one might think this would be a nonissue, as the students are always in the presence of the teacher in the classroom. However, the supervision plan must cover the out-of-classroom situations. For example, if the playground that the children use for recess or PE is a large area, arrangements must be made to ensure that the child who has demonstrated sexual behavior problems is always within immediate eyesight of the teacher. Additionally, all bathroom activities should be done separately from other children. Such a strict plan puts a burden of responsibility on teachers and aides. Therefore, teachers should be repeatedly consulted so that they can report how the plan is working and have the opportunity to suggest adaptations that will better fit their classroom schedule or request additional support. Teachers should be encouraged to modify the plan and decrease the level of supervision if the child improves his/her impulse control, displays better behavior at school and home, and goes an extended period of time without inappropriate sexual behavior.

Helping the Child to Maintain Appropriate Behavior

In addition to supervision, there are other ways that teachers can support children's efforts to extinguish their sexual behavior problems. For example, teachers should be encouraged in their efforts to remove anything from the classroom that might be sexually stimulating. This may include teachers' being attentive to, but not tolerating, inappropriate sexual innuendoes, jokes, or cursing from any student. Any physical or even verbal aggression should be monitored, as it may be sexually stimulating to the child (Johnson, 1990). Children with a history of sexual behavior problems must be most at risk for repeated difficulties during quiet or unstructured times as fantasies or disturbing feelings may escalate during these periods (Gil & Johnson, 1993; Johnson, 1990). Finally, teachers should be aware of the potential that their own clothing and behaviors may be interpreted in a sexualized way and raise anxiety for children with histories of sexual victimization and/or sexual behavior problems (Slater & Gallagher, 1989).

Addressing children's sexual behavior problems can be an uncomfortable role for teachers. With the needed information and support from school professionals, however, they can be a valuable influence in this role.

False Allegations against Teachers

One additional emotionally charged topic for teachers is the fear of false allegations. Concerns in this area are common. In one survey 24% of teachers indicated that they were aware of allegations of abuse having been made against a teacher in their school district within the past year and 56% aware of similar allegations within the past several years. In this sample, 37% were worried about being falsely accused during the course of doing their job (Anderson & Levine, 1999).

In responding to the vignettes in this survey, teachers with more experience were more likely to advise against being alone in a room with a student, and against touching or hugging a student (Anderson & Levine, 1999). While some degree of caution regarding these matters is understandable, an overly protective stance is not without costs. "To the extent that fears about allegations cause teaches to limit contact with their students, there are potentially negative consequences within the teaching environment" (Anderson & Levine, 1999, p. 842)

Anderson and Levine (1999) go on to detail the costs of an overly protective stance. First, there may be a decrease in teachers identifying abuse victims. Teachers who do not maintain close enough relationships are likely the recipients of fewer disclosures and may not observe closely enough to notice physical indicators. Second, students may be denied some of the special opportunities for positive growth experiences that can occur in an educational setting. This may be especially unfortunate for students who have abusive or neglectful parents, as these students do not have opportunities for such positive relationships outside of school (Anderson & Levine, 1999).

Tower (1992) notes that often, years after their abuse, "survivors" often name teachers as among the most positively influential people in their lives. To have teachers "back off" in a way that misses the positive opportunities would be a great cost to all students, but particularly to those most in need. A reasonable degree of caution is certainly appropriate. For example, students not being invited to teachers' homes or not spending extensive time alone after school with a teacher may be policies that schools adopt or that individual teachers choose. Avoiding all personal relationships or physical contact with students, however, is probably an overly conservative reaction to potential, yet improbable, dangers.

In sum, teachers have an absolutely critical role to play in responding to children who have been victims of maltreatment. Teachers, therefore, need and deserve the support of school-based mental health professionals in identifying and reporting child abuse and neglect. Additionally, teachers may benefit from information and support in responding to the parents and the students after making any oral report. Finally, special topics such as sexual behavior problems and teachers' concerns about false allegations about themselves are worthy of special attention from the school's professionals.

PARTNERING WITH PARENTS

Although teachers definitely have a significant role to play in the lives of their students, the even more influential role of parents cannot be overestimated. For a child who has been maltreated, this is even more likely the case. Thus, for mental health practitioners, consulting with teachers is certainly a critical role; however, developing healthy partnership and collaborations with parents may make an even greater difference in the lives of children who have been abused. Any positive influence on parents of children who have been abused or neglected, any support or consultation offered, may indirectly—but strongly—support the recovery of a child who has been maltreated.

In recent years, there has been a movement in school psychology and related fields toward increasing active collaboration between the school and the home, and a greater tendency to view parents as partners. Christenson (1995) has pointed out that home–school collaboration is more than an activity—rather, it is an attitude. "It occurs when parents and educators share common goals, are seen as equals, and both contribute to the process" (p. 253). This same collaborative attitude should apply in working with parents whose children have been abused (Tharinger & Horton, 1992). Parents and educators can work together for the best interests of the child who has been abused. Certainly, parents whose children have been abused may need support and information from the school. At the same time, in most cases, parents have much to offer as well. They are experts on their own children.

Guidelines for developing home–school collaborations have been described (Christenson, 1995). Clearly these apply, and perhaps are even more important to remain mindful of when working with families of abused children. Two seem especially important.

A Belief in Shared Responsibility

Both the home and the school have important roles and responsibilities in a child's development. While this notion has important implications for academic success, it is critical as it relates to child maltreatment as well. Both home and school have an obligation to keep children safe when in their care, to do all they can to prevent children from being abused. If school personnel or parents become aware that a child may have been abused or neglected, it is their responsibility to take appropriate action to protect the child. A sense of shared responsibility is equally important in supporting the emotional well-being of a child who is already known to have been maltreated. For example, it is the responsibility of schools to notice, respond to, and discuss with parents any evidence of ongoing distress, behavior problems, or other aspects of the aftermath of abuse. Schools also have a responsibility to offer what services they can to support the recovery of children who have been abused and to make referrals for those needed services they cannot provide. It is the responsibility of parents to do what they can to respond to information about their children's distress, to be supportive by being physically and psychological available to their children—who may have extra needs (Tharinger, 1991)—and to secure additional resources, as needed.

The general home–school collaboration literature has described that "talking down," or patronizing parents, is an obstacle to the desired sense of shared responsibility (Christenson, 1995). If school practitioners want working partnerships with parents in the response to child maltreatment, they must treat parents as partners.

The Importance of Taking the Other's Perspective

School personnel should seek to empathize with the parents' experience. While important in general, this guideline is critical to the development of partnerships with parents after their children have been abused. Each must understand the other party.

As discussed earlier, most nonoffending parents—such as mothers of children who have been sexually abused or "battered women" whose children have been exposed to domestic violence—do not fit the stereotype of an uncaring, unavailable parent. Instead, these women are often doing the best they can under extraordinarily difficult circumstances (Lyon, 1999).

School mental health practitioners seeking to develop collaborative relationships with parents are reminded of the numerous stressors that these parents face, even if they have left the offending partner. Certainly, there is the overwhelming emotional anguish of accepting that a partner betrayed one's trust and harmed one's child. Many women have their own PTSD reactions, perhaps in part because, in addition to the immediate stressor, this event brings back memories and reactions to their own abuse history (Famularo et al., 1994; Tharinger, 1991). Safety concerns for themselves and their children might still be a major issue (Edleson, 1999). Often there are ongoing legal stressors (abuse trials, divorce matters, custody disputes), financial pressures, and time demands. Parents have frequently had to move, have lost relationships with key support figures, and have had increasing dilemmas regarding the need to work to support the family and the need to spend time with their children (Lyon, 1999). Once a school-based clinician considers the heavy weight on the shoulders of these parents, it is much easier to be accommodating regarding scheduling conferences, patient when parents have not yet followed up on a referral, and understanding when a note or call goes unanswered.

Parents, likewise, must understand the perspective of the school. At times, this may need to be directly explained. Teachers typically do care about each child in their class, especially those with particular needs (including an abuse history), but teachers are frequently seeking to educate, and socialize, 30 or more children at once. In upper grades, the teacher likely has six classes of 30. Thus, parents, too, must be patient with teachers who cannot immediately return every call, spend extensive time with every child, or be accommodating to one in a way that causes all others to sacrifice. School psychologists, counselors, and social workers may need to assist parents in empathizing with the teachers' position and in finding others who can offer needed extra support. Additionally, parents must understand that, while school personnel want to be compassionate and patient with children who are acting out in response to the abuse, schools must be kept safe for all children. School personnel will need parents' assistance in addressing emotional and behavioral problems so that the children who have experienced abuse can be supported in making positive changes and the peers around those children will not be victimized. Parents should be encouraged to assist schools in problem solving particular situations. For example, in one situation, a parent was upset with the school for having her child, a victim of sexual abuse, assigned to detention with only one male supervisor. While the parent did not object to the detention due to her child's misbehavior, she felt the supervisory arrangements would put her daughter at risk for feeling uncomfortable, at least, and being revictimized, at worst. While there might be some speculation that the mother's concerns might have risen to the level of paranoia, her protective instincts should be honored. If, rather than attacking the school, the mother could affirm her support of the school's position regarding her child's misbehavior, share her concerns, and suggest alternative arrangements (e.g., the mother could come to school during detention; her daughter could serve a before-school detention in the school office with a female teacher as supervisor; etc.), the school could likely make accommodations.

These two assumptions—that the response to children who have been abused or neglected is a shared responsibility between home and school and that each must honor the other's perspective—are important foundations in consulting with parents. These should form the philosophical basis for parent consultation on these matters.

Moving from the philosophical to the pragmatic, a number of principles apply to daily best-practice.

1. *Contact with parents should be welcomed, not avoided.* School mental health professionals, like teachers, might be tempted to avoid contact with families once abuse has been reported. However, again, it is critical to remember that

such a response may be detrimental to the child. Supporting parents—whatever the circumstances—is a way of supporting the maltreated child. Nonoffending parents often do not fit the stereotypes that have arisen. Furthermore, parents who do happen to be stressed out, overburdened, or ill equipped for their roles are all the more deserving of caring, nonjudgmental support, just as their children deserve protection when needed (Gelardo & Sanford, 1987).

2. *Process and content matter.* Parents, like teachers, may benefit from mental health consultations with and general supportive relationships with school-based clinicians. Particularly during the initial postdisclosure, or discovery crisis stage, their need may be evident, as even nonoffending parents feel overwhelmed, inadequate, and guilty. Certainly parents' own issues of flashbacks, anger, and depression will influence their parenting. Later, the general support of school-based clinicians may be appreciated as parents need the encouragement to persevere to cooperate with the CPS system, follow through on referrals for needed resources, and to continue to seek to balance self-care and child-care needs through what may be a long journey. But, just as teachers need not only supportive mental health consultations but also information, skills, and resources, so it is with parents. The school-based mental health professional can offer needed "content" as well as a sensitive "process."

3. *Parents should be helped to understand and respond to children's behaviors.* One of the key topics on which parents need information is why their children are acting as they do. "Why is my child so angry with me? I wasn't the one who hit him?" "Why is my child so scared of school? She was never hurt there." "When will these nightmares end?" "What should I do when my child runs away?" Parents may benefit from "a lay person's" explanation of a number of the theoretical explanations described in the teacher's section earlier in this chapter. Additionally, a number of the practical suggestions for teachers (e.g., be patient, change takes time, be compassionate but still correct the behaviors, etc.) are good advice for parents, as well. Having books available (e.g., *When Your Child Has Been Molested: A Parent's Guide to Healing and Recovery* (Hagans & Case, 1988) may be useful, and appreciated by, many parents.

For parents, though, there are the additional, more personal, questions that need to be answered and quite possibly distorted thinking that needs to be corrected. For example, when Debbie received a call notifying her that her son, Dustin had been the apparent aggressor in a fight on the playground, she broke into tears and stated to the school psychologist that her son acts "just like" his abusive father (the mother's ex-husband), that he must be "destined" to be an abuser. While this thinking is (at best) understandable, it is likely not accurate, obviously an obstacle to a healthy mother–son relationship, and potentially grist for a self-fulfilling prophecy. While a family counselor may provide more intensive interventions with Debbie and Dustin later, school clinicians may be the first to begin to suggest other ways Debbie could view the situation. By combining mental health consultation with valuable information, the school psychologist may help the mother understand that, while there are some similarities, her son is not her "ex," that certainly he may have learned to be aggressive from his father, but he might also be acting out his feelings about all that has gone on in the family. With needed help, the son can learn to manage his anger and have a healthy nonviolent life.

Beyond understanding the behaviors, parents need to know how to respond to their children's acting out. Parents must understand that the goal must be reduce the distress and anxiety in their home. Thus, parents should avoid yelling, hitting, or threatening the child with rejection or punishment (Friedrich, 1995). Instead, corrective help should be proffered in the form of natural and logical consequences, carried out in a consistent way, in the context of a secure relationship. The parent's message to the child essentially must be "There are some behaviors that are not acceptable. There will be consequences when you make those choices. I will get you help so that you can learn to make other choices. And most importantly, no matter what, I still love you."

Parents whose children are demonstrating sexual behavior problems may need specific assistance and suggestions. Parents should be urged not to overreact or underreact, as neither response is likely helpful. Depending on the severity of the problems, two responses are likely most important: securing specialized counseling services and providing adequate supervision. Such literature, as the book *Children Who Molest: A Guide for Parents of Young Sex Offenders* (Gil, 1987) may be useful to recommend or provide to parents.

4. *Parents should be encouraged to seek needed additional resources.* As we noted in Chapter 4, helping parents furnish additional services for their children may be extremely important. Severe traumatic responses or specific difficulties such as sexual behavior problems may best be addressed by a specialist in the community. In addition to seeking therapy for their children, parents may need encouragement to seek counseling for themselves. Parents may be overwhelmed, experiencing their own posttraumatic stress, or feeling intense anger or confusion in response to their child's current functioning. General parenting classes may be helpful, but parents may need more intensive, specialized services, depending on the family's power dynamics. As Friedrich (1995, p. 76) points out, just "Sending parents to parent training because they hate their child will not aid them in liking him more or having more compassion for him or his hurts. They may learn some new strategies but unless they are committed and attuned to their son, they are likely to use these new strategies coercively with him." Groups for parents whose children have been abused and/or individual counseling for the parent(s) may be helpful.

5. *Parents should be urged to find that delicate balance of self-care and child care.* While juggling roles and needs is a challenging task for all parents, for those whose children have been maltreated, the balancing act is intensified. The children may have intense needs, and in many ways need their parents to "be there for them." On the other hand, in many situations, the parents are undergoing enormous stress simultaneously and are in great need of self-care. As school clinicians have opportunities to consult with parents, they can help them to see that these are not necessarily separate issues but can be met and dealt with simultaneously. For example, children need their parents, but they need a parent who is not depressed (Tharinger, 1991). Thus, honestly addressing one's own issues simultaneously does not necessarily take away from, but rather helps, one's children in the long run. By modeling self-care, additionally, parents are helping their child. On a daily basis, for example, parents can teach their children affect regulation. "You know, I have had a hard day, and I feel kind of stressed and nervous inside. I am going to go take a hot bath, and then I'll be back to read you your stories." "Jason, Mommy is getting frustrated and a little angry right now. I'm going to take a little break, take a few deep breaths, and then I'll come right back and we'll work something out." By taking care of oneself, and articulating the process, parents are also taking care of their children.

6. *Parents should be encouraged to do what they can to prevent any future abuse.* Children who have been abused are at risk for revictimization. Parents should be encouraged to do what they can to help inoculate their children. Johnson (1999), in her book *Understanding Your Child's Sexual Behavior: What's Natural and Healthy* (another helpful reading suggestion for parents), makes a number of specific recommendations. Children, Johnson argues, are most at risk if they do not know what is natural and healthy. Therefore, parents are urged to help teach children boundaries, ownership, and personal space through a variety of day-to-day opportunities. For example, parents are encouraged to respect a child's request that tickling stop. Children should also be allowed to have their own toys or their own space that is respected. Parents should also model their own healthy boundaries.

Additionally, parents' protective instincts should be encouraged (Daro, 1994; Wurtele, 1998). Parents must remember that children, including those who have already been abused, are at greatest risk for being abused by someone known to the family. Parents should be aware that predatory offenders often will ingratiate themselves with parents first in order to gain access to a child. Thus, without allowing paranoia to arise, parents should be encouraged in their efforts to appropriately monitor their child's contact with others. Most important of all is maintaining a close relationship with one's child so that, should the need arise, a child would immediately disclose if abuse occurred or even if he/she were uncomfortable with someone's behavior toward him/her. Children should be directly told that it would be OK to tell parents about any such situations—even if they occurred with someone known to, or in, the family.

Parental monitoring of children's Internet access and use is also wise, as increasing numbers of children are being solicited through this medium (Finkelhor et al., 2000). Parents should be aware of their children's or adolescents' use of the Internet and should consider using filters or antipornography screens to prevent unwanted sexual and/or predatory contact.

7. *Parents should be encouraged to view their child as more than a victim.* Consultation with parents should discourage denial or minimization of their child's victimization history or need for protection; however, overemphasizing the abuse aspect of a child's life is also not helpful. Children who have been maltreated should be viewed as children first. In most cases, parents should encourage them to participate in a full range of healthy activities and experiences, allowing them to gain a variety of experiences. Having children more involved in therapy activities (e.g., group counseling one night, individual therapy the next, family sessions another day) and not having time for sports, clubs, or informal social activities with their peers may be counterproductive. Parents should be encouraged that their child's victimization experience is one significant experience in his/her history, one that may need to be processed and integrated, but it is not all of his/her history, and it is not all of who he/she is. Parents need to have the opportunity to be "just parents" and let their kids be "just kids."

CONCLUSION

Clearly, the overwhelming influence that parents have on their child's life cannot be overemphasized. They need the support to fulfill these roles in a way that promotes their children's recovery. School practitioners can be an important part of that support. By consulting with, providing information to, and generally supporting teachers and parents, school-based clinicians help to create a therapeutic setting in which a child who has been victimized can avoid revictimization and go on to live a healthy life.

In-Service Training Overhead 1.
Definitions of Child Abuse and Neglect

Physical abuse

- Physical abuse is an act of commission by a parent or caretaker characterized by the infliction of physical injury.
- May result from extended physical altercations (e.g., hitting, kicking, shaking).
- Or brief, isolated incidents (e.g., being burned, thrown down stairs, bitten, poisoned).

Sexual abuse

- Sexual abuse is "the involvement of dependent, developmentally immature children in sexual activities that they do not fully comprehend and therefore to which they are unable to give informed consent and/or which violate the taboos of society" (Krugman & Jones, 1987, p. 286).
- May involve contact (e.g., fondling and intercourse).
- May not involve contact (e.g., involvement in pornography, voyeurism).

Emotional abuse

- Emotional abuse consists of the repeated acts and/or omissions of parents or caregivers in meeting the child's emotional needs.
- Includes treating a child in a way that is rejecting, degrading, terrorizing, isolating, corrupting, exploiting, or denying emotional responsiveness.

Neglect

- Neglect has been defined as a form of maltreatment characterized by a chronic lack of care.
- May be physical, emotional, or educational.

Exposure to domestic violence

- Children are frequently unintended victims.

In-Service Training Overhead 2.
Incidence and Prevalence of Child Abuse and Neglect

Over 3 million children are reported to be abused or neglected each year. Over 1 million cases are substantiated. Many more occur. Reported rates represent the "tip of the iceberg."

Physical abuse

- 16–19% of adults report being physically abused in their childhood.

Sexual abuse

- Approximately 15–20% of females and 5–10% of males report being sexually abused before age 18.

Emotional abuse

- Difficult to estimate.
- Many families have some degree of emotional abuse.

Neglect

- Difficult to estimate.
- Represents 50+% of child protective services reports.

Exposure to domestic violence

- Approximately 15% of adults report childhood exposure.

Note. Often victims experience multiple forms of maltreatment.

In-Service Training Overhead 3.
Possible Effects of Child Abuse and Neglect

Note. These symptoms do not necessarily indicate abuse, as most may have multiple origins; however, these are examples of commonly noted symptoms in children who have been victimized.

Physical
- Injuries
- Somatic complaints
- Failure to thrive
- Physical injuries (e.g., suspicious bruises, welts, broken bones)

Emotional
- Depression
- Anxiety
- Fear
- Hopelessness
- Anger

Behavioral
- Internalizing (e.g., withdrawal)
- Externalizing (e.g., aggression, bullying)
- Sexual behavior problems

Cognitive
- Damaged goods syndrome
- Learned helplessness
- Identification with perpetrator

In-Service Training Overhead 4.
Mediators of the Effects of Child Maltreatment

Child Characteristics

- Age at onset of the abuse or neglect
- Gender
- Level of cognitive functioning

Preabuse family functioning

- Quality of the parent–child relationship
- Emotional climate of the family
- The child's emotional/mental health functioning

Aspects of the abuse experience

- Severity
- Chronicity
- Exposure to multiple forms of maltreatment
- Biological and/or emotional relationship with the offender
- Level of threat or force involved
- Response to disclosure

Coping strategies/cognitive interpretation

- Type of coping strategies used (i.e., problem-focused vs. emotion-focused)
- Powerlessness/learned helplessness
- Attribution of responsibility (i.e., self-blame vs. blaming offender)

In-Service Training Overhead 5.
Reporting Abuse

◆ Rationale

Legal: Teachers are mandated reporters.

Ethical: Professional.

Moral: Caring response to children.

◆ Only "reason to suspect" is required.

◆ Protected for "good-faith reports."

In-Service Training Overhead 6.
Making a Report

Gather essential facts

- Child's name and contact information

- Suspected abuse

- Reason for suspicion (as detailed as possible)

- Details (including quotes of child's disclosure)

- Suspected perpetrator's name and contact information

- Information regarding parents

Call child protective services _____ if suspected perpetrator is a parent or caregiver.

Call Police or Sheriff's Dept. _____if suspected perpetrator is not a caregiver or parent.

Inform the principal.

In-Service Training Overhead 7.
Obstacles to Reporting

Fears

- Imagine how the child feels.

- Isn't protecting the child worth doing what needs to be done?

Lack of information or expertise

- Only need to suspect.

- Call CPS if you have questions.

School-based

- The principal is not the "gatekeeper."

- *You* are the mandated reporter.

Concerns regarding child protective services

- Reluctance to getting the child in "The System."

- To not report doesn't give the child a chance.

- Speak with a supervisor as needed.

CHAPTER 7

♦♦♦

Prevention in the Schools

♦

A frequently told story to emphasize the need for prevention is that of a town where there were a number of drownings. One day, a few caring townspeople, hearing distressed voices, ran to the river to help. In a few hours of hard work, they had pulled many would-be drowning vicitims to safety, but their work was not yet done. Many more people seemed to be floating downstream, struggling to survive in the rough water. The frantic townspeople called for more help, became more organized, and worked harder and harder at pulling more people out of the river. Finally, one of the rescuers started walking away from the others. "What are you doing?" the others yelled angrily. "There are others who need to be rescued. Don't you care?" "Yes, I care," he answered. "I care enough to go upstream and see if I can fix whatever is causing people to fall in."

The efforts of school professionals to identify, report, and intervene with child maltreatment are certainly warranted and commendable; however, these actions are aimed at pulling children out of "the river" of abuse and neglect after they have already been immersed and, in some cases, nearly drowned. Individuals, schools, communities, and society at large must also focus on the point at which children are entering "the river," to make long-term strides in the prevention of child maltreatment. This chapter will describe three levels of prevention and discuss how schools may be involved at each level, including victimization prevention programs and their effectiveness. Finally, key components to be considered by school professionals when developing and implementing a child maltreatment prevention program will be presented.

THEORETICAL UNDERSTANDING OF ETIOLOGY

Child maltreatment is a complex phenomenon. Its prevention demands a complex solution. Selecting an approach to prevention may depend upon one's theoretical understanding of the etiology of maltreatment. In other words, deciding how to prevent abuse is based on what one believes causes it. There are numerous risk factors (e.g., individual child or parent characteristics, family dynamics, cultural influences) indicated in the cause of maltreatment and identified as protective factors that may mediate the onset or impact of maltreatment (see Chapter 1 for a review). Ecological models that emphasize the interactions of these factors provide the broadest understanding of maltreatment and highlight the importance of prevention at multiple levels (Holden & Nabors, 1999). However, the diversity of risk factors creates many challenges in preparing a comprehensive prevention program. An additional challenge in the prevention of child maltreatment is the requirement of complex behavior change by many individuals to ensure preventative efforts are transactional and cut across ecological contexts (Holden & Nabors, 1999).

In light of these obstacles, great gains have been made in the prevention of child maltreatment during the past three decades, with several model programs being developed. Some of these programs have been aimed at reducing the risk of further abuse or neglect, while others focus on stopping the occurrence of maltreatment even before it is fully manifested.

LEVELS OF PREVENTION

Further delineation of prevention activities results in three levels differentiated by their target audience (see Table 7.1). Primary or universal prevention activities are aimed at the general population in order to prevent the onset of new cases of child maltreatment (Cosentino, 1989; Holden & Nabors, 1999; Newman & Lutzker, 1990). These programs usually target environmental or community factors influencing maltreatment (e.g., poverty, teen pregnancy, substance abuse). Primary or universal prevention does not target any particular group, so participation at this level is reportedly less stigmatizing (Greenberg, Domitrovitch, & Bumbarger, 1999). Some examples might include the national media campaign for shaken baby syndrome, the Drug Abuse Resistance Education (DARE) prevention program provided by police, school-based sexual abuse prevention programs, and community parent education programs. Disadvantages or shortcomings of these types of programs are (1) the messages often are too general or vague that those who need most to understand them or change go unaffected; (2) their effectiveness is often difficult to assess; and (3) much of the effort may be expended on individuals who are unlikely to be either the victim or the perpetrator of child maltreatment (Greenberg et al., 1999; Holden & Nabors, 1999).

Secondary or selected prevention activities are directed toward individuals or communities with a higher incidence of maltreatment risk factors

TABLE 7.1. Levels of Prevention

Level	Description	Community examples	School examples
Primary/universal	Addresses the population as a whole to increase understanding and reporting of child maltreatment	Media campaigns Public service announcements Crisis hotlines Parent education programs Community support groups Big Brothers/Big Sisters mentoring programs	Health and sex education courses School sexual/physical abuse programs Schoolwide problem-solving or conflict resolution programs
Secondary/selective	Targets at-risk individuals or subgroups to stop the occurrence of child maltreatment	Respite care facilities Family support/parental competency programs Home visitation programs—for first-time or young parents	High school life education programs Preschool programs School meal programs Before- and after-school care programs
Tertiary/indicated	Provides services to victims, perpetrators, and families to prevent negative effects, further abuse, and to reduce the impact of child maltreatment	Individual therapy—for child or offender Group therapy—for child or offender Clinic-based family therapy In-home family preservation services Required parent education—for families involved with CPS Domestic violence emergency shelters	School-based social skills, anger management, or self-esteem enhancement groups Individual counseling Topic-focused group counseling Individual education plans

Note. Information for this table was obtained from the following sources: Daro (1994); Greenberg, Domitrovich, and Bumbarger (1999); Holden and Nabors (1999); Marion (1982); and National Clearinghouse on Child Abuse and Neglect Information (2000).

(e.g., poverty, parental substance abuse, young parents, children or parents with disabilities) (Greenberg et al., 1999; Holden & Nabors, 1999; National Clearinghouse on Child Abuse and Neglect Information, 2000). These programs focus on early identification of, and resource provision to, at-risk families before maltreatment occurs (Newman & Lutzker, 1990). By targeting risk and protective factors, multiple negative outcomes can be addressed, creating a more cost-effective approach (Greenberg et al., 1999). Family life education programs for pregnant teens, school meal programs, respite care for families with children with special needs, home visitation programs for first-time or young parents, and support groups for parents or children are all examples designed to prevent the spread of maltreatment.

Tertiary or indicated prevention is the provision of services to individuals or families after abuse or neglect has already occurred (Cosentino, 1989; Holden & Nabors, 1999). These efforts are designed to prevent further abuse or neglect and to minimize the negative consequences of maltreatment. Therapeutic services at this level may be provided to the child, perpetrator, or family. Intensive, in-home family preservation services, social skills training for children, and sexual offender or domestic violence groups are just a few of the many types of prevention at this level. Short-term interventions produce time-limited benefits, whereas comprehensive programs are more likely to create lasting benefits (Greenberg et al., 1999). This may be due in part to the difficulty in changing the thoughts and actions of others but also to the length of the cycle of maltreatment (Holden & Nabors, 1999). Thus, tertiary or indicated prevention activities are the most costly. However, they could be drastically reduced if efforts at the other levels were better able to stop the progression of child maltreatment.

THE ROLE OF SCHOOLS

Schools are the largest institution with regular daily access to children over an extended time period. For some of these children, school is a sanctuary where they can come early, stay late, and thereby hide from the abuses of the outside world or their home situation. Because of this, many teachers and counselors have information gained from observations, or received directly from children, that no one else has (Morgan, 1994). Additionally, schools are the site, second only to the home setting, where the most social learning takes place (Wolfe & Jaffe, 1999). It is this unique position that makes schools an ideal place for prevention activities necessary to change the attitudes and behaviors of children (Greenberg et al., 1999).

Schools have been involved in promoting the overall well-being of children, and thus prevention, in numerous ways for many years. Schools may be spurring a number of prevention initiatives that may never have been thought of as such. For example, specific services (e.g., special education services, occupational therapy, physical therapy, speech and language therapy) for children with special needs, reduced-price lunches and breakfast programs, before- and after-school care programs, policies against corporal punishment, a chance for positive experiences through achievement and interpersonal relationships, and healthy role models who provide consistent care and support (Broadhurst, 1980) are actually prevention efforts.

It was not until recently that schools began to formally recognize and intentionally play a role in child maltreatment prevention. By the 1980s schools also took an active role in the prevention of child sexual abuse by providing personal safety and victimization prevention programs to children. In the last decade, a majority of schools (85%) have been found to offer such programs, with over half (64%) of the programs being mandated by the states (Daro, 1994). Further, in a national phone survey, 67% of children between the ages of 10 and 16 reported having participated in such a prevention program and 95% said they would recommend the program to other children (Finkelhor & Dziuba-Leatherman, 1995). Parents, teachers, and administrators have also found these programs to be helpful and important (Abrahams et al., 1992; Daro, 1994; Finkelhor & Dziuba-Leatherman, 1995; Wurtele, 1998). School-based victimization prevention programs are the most likely forums through which the majority of children may be reached. They are also an ideal setting because they allow for ongoing discussions and reinforcement of the content even after the program is completed (Rispens, Aleman, & Goudena, 1997).

Schools, however, are encouraged to take an even broader role in prevention efforts. Schools have staff with expertise and training in a diversity of areas and have physical facilities that can be used beyond the regular school hours (Tower, 1992). Schools can become central locations, or the "hub of the community," at which expanded prevention efforts can take place. This is not to suggest that school personnel have to be the only ones involved in the prevention programs or that staff would be expected to venture outside their competencies. Rather, schools have the potential to provide fully integrated prevention models by collaborating with the community and capitalizing on the resources the schools already possess (Greenberg et al., 1999).

THE ROLE OF THE SCHOOL-BASED
MENTAL HEALTH PRACTITIONER

School psychologists, counselors, and social workers have been identified as the key personnel likely to lead the school's response to child maltreatment (Batchelor, Dean, Gridley, & Batchelor, 1990; Cosentino, 1989; Holden & Nabors, 1999; Horton, 1995; James & Burch, 1999; Tharinger, Russian, & Robinson, 1989; Vevier & Tharinger, 1986). These school-based mental health practitioners have the opportunity to be involved in all three levels of prevention.

Primary Prevention

Schools can be involved in prevention in multiple ways. Seeking to provide others with information and developing programs that will address the general risk factors of child maltreatment (e.g., parent education) are examples of primary prevention.

Information Providers

In order for schools to be involved with prevention, everyone—including nurses, teachers, and even superintendents—must be made aware of child maltreatment. They need to have knowledge of the rates of occurrence, risk and protective factors, and the negative consequences of each subtype. School-based practitioners can provide this information through in-service training and ongoing consultation with personnel. This information may also be provided to parents and the community through workshops and presentations at area group meetings (e.g., United Way, YMCA Childcare Programs, the Women's League). Knowledge of maltreatment is needed by administrators, parents, and community members to understand and support other prevention efforts, especially school-based programs (Cosentino, 1989).

In order to serve as an informed prevention resource to their school and community, school-based practitioners will need to stay abreast of the research and treatment of child abuse and neglect. This may include reading, attending workshops, or completing a university course (Vevier & Tharinger, 1986). It may also mean establishing and maintaining professional and social networks to obtain support for their endeavors (Vevier & Tharinger, 1986). It is not uncommon for school practitioners who are trying to lead their schools into broader prevention programs to be faced with resistance from educators and parents who believe prevention is important but do not want schools to play a central role (see Table 7.2 for common concerns raised by parents and teachers). Practitioners should keep in mind that school personnel and community members need repeated exposure to this information in order to be able to work with affected children and families effectively.

Parent Education

School-based mental health professionals may provide parent education programs both on site and in the community. The knowledge these practitioners have in the areas of child development, learning, and behavior modification, along with their daily interactions with children, makes them valuable re-

TABLE 7.2. Common Concerns Expressed by Parents and Teachers Regarding Prevention Programs in Schools

Concern	Points for response or follow-up questions
"The curriculum is already too crowded, and I can't move anything else off the list to cover this issue."	◆ Child maltreatment prevention is essential, and children may not receive it otherwise. ◆ Prevention issues can be incorporated into current subject matters. ◆ Long-term benefits would certainly outweigh short-term costs.
"I don't want to know the specifics about maltreatment and reporting, because then I may have to make a report and go to court. What if I am wrong? What if the parent gets angry?"	◆ Educators are *mandated* reporters. ◆ Awareness of indicators and reporting procedures may alleviate fears. ◆ Legally protected if report is in good faith. ◆ Ongoing consultation and support will be provided by school-based practitioners. ◆ Without your involvement, children are left to suffer.
"It is not the role of the school to teach sex education and parenting skills. These children should learn this information at home, and I think most parents are talking to their kids about sex."	◆ Parents and schools should work collaboratively to prevent maltreatment. ◆ Both parents and schools may assume the other is providing this information, and yet children fail to receive it. ◆ Schools can provide parents with accurate, age-appropriate information in these areas. ◆ Sexual abuse prevention programs focus on personal safety, not necessarily sex education.
"This type of prevention program will only make my child afraid of me or encourage him to call 911 every time he gets a spanking or I give him a bath."	◆ While some children may feel worried, the majority feel safer and more competent after the programs. ◆ A slightly stressful reaction may not indicate a negative effect but an understanding.
or	
"I don't want my child to be afraid of everyone she meets. She already has a hard time sleeping."	◆ Prevention programs educate children about good, bad, and secretive touches. ◆ Parental involvement in prevention programs increases understanding and alleviates some concerns.

Note. Information for this table was obtained from the following sources: Cosentino (1989) and Sudermann, Jaffe, and Hastings (1995).

sources to parents. Although there are numerous risk factors for maltreatment, many are related to parents and the parent–child attachment. It is not strangers in prison for heineous crimes that communities should fear harming children, but the people they know and see regularly (Foxhall, 2000). Recall from Chapter 1 that most offenders are either a parent or a person already known to the child. The long-term solution is not, however, through the judicial system. Rather, school personnel should take a supportive and educational role with all parents. The goal should be to increase parental competence. It is not enough to just educate parents as to the wrongfulness and harmfulness of child maltreatment. Practitioners must give parents skills to replace the (in)actions that they are asking them to eliminate from their thinking. One can hardly expect parents to readily give up the only method of "discipline" they know without teaching them an effective alternative. School practitioners can also provide parents with training in self-care and coping strategies and help connect them to resources for ongoing support. Additionally, increasing parents' protective instincts should be a goal. Frequently, parents of children who were abused by a neighbor or relative subsequently reflect that they sensed something was not right and that they should have trusted their instincts. Practitioners can encourage parents to be more responsive to their own protective instincts.

Life Skills Training

Schools have also begun to implement general prevention programs for children and adolescents. Many of these programs include training in social skills (i.e., how to meet one's needs through interactions with others), affective education (i.e., the identification and appropriate expression of emotions, and empathy training), and problem solving and coping skills (e.g., steps in decision making, methods of problem-focused coping, impulse control, and conflict resolution). School-based mental health practitioners are often the ones who select and implement these programs on a schoolwide scale. Practitioners may also train teachers to provide instruction on these programs, to reinforce the concepts and skills on a daily basis. Administrative support in the form of dollars and resources (e.g., planning time, supplies, paid training days) will help ensure greater success with these programs.

In the secondary schools family life education programs are aimed at teaching all adolescents daily living skills and preparation for parenting (Marion, 1982; Tower, 1992). These activities may occur as part of the established curriculum or through special programs. For example, budgeting or investing may be taught as part of a consumer education course, while time management and work-study skills may be addressed across the curriculum. School practitioners may be asked to advise on curriculum choice in any of these areas, but are more commonly consulted on the selection of health and sex education curricula. More comprehensive curricula that focus on child and adolescent development (given the broad age for the onset of puberty), normal sexuality, reproduction, sexually transmitted diseases, and sexual responsibility should be selected or created by drawing relevant material from numerous sources.

Parent preparation classes may encompass a broad array of issues pertinent to interpersonal relationships and ultimately parenthood. For example, gender inequality, sex role stereotypes, and attitudes about violence may be debated, along with direct instruction on age-appropriate expectations for children, child guidance strategies, and cultural factors contributing to abuse (Marion, 1982; Sudermann, Jaffe, & Hastings, 1995). These programs should include information tailored to the children's developmental level; the most effective programs include fewer lectures and more dialoging about students' personal feelings and concerns (Marion, 1982; Wolfe & Jaffe, 1999). School practitioners may need to use this information if asked to advise on curriculum or the approach to take in teaching this type of content. An even greater role for practitioners may be to consult with teachers regarding specific observations, discussions, or disclosures that may arise in such a course.

Personal Safety and Victimization Prevention

Finally, at the primary level of prevention school-based practitioners may be asked to assist in the selection and implementation of decision-making and problem-solving strategies to decrease the vulnerability of children to abuse or neglect, or attendant consequences (Cosentino, 1989; James & Burch, 1999). In the past these have most commonly been programs targeting personal safety and victimization prevention. However, a better understanding of the risk and protective factors associated with all types of maltreatment and the more recent school violence incidents have prompted more programs on such general topics as bullying, conflict resolution, and violence in dating relationships.

The knowledge and training school-based practitioners have in maltreatment, child development, and child evaluation will serve to assist schools or districts in choosing the most cost-effective prevention program (Batchelor et al., 1990; Vevier & Tharinger, 1986). Effective communication and leadership skills are prime requirements for practitioners as they attempt to organize and direct prevention planning committees (Cosentino, 1989). It is these planning committees, and not the practitioners alone, who will evaluate and determine the specific components of a school prevention program. However, maltreatment prevention is a rapidly growing field, and practitioners are encouraged to keep up with the most recent research on the programs that have been developed and their relative efficaciousness.

Given the integral role that schools have played in child sexual abuse prevention and the important function that practitioners serve in selecting and implementing such programs, it seems appropriate to more closely examine these programs and their effectiveness. There are a variety of sexual abuse prevention programs developed for both preschool and school-aged children. These curricula vary in length (i.e., some extending over several weeks or months, others lasting only a single day) and presentation medium (e.g., lectures, panel discussions, videos, comic books, role-plays, worksheets). The four primary goals common to most programs are to (1) educate children to the warning signs of abusive situations, along with the distinctions between appropriate and inappropriate touching; (2) teach them strategies for stopping abuse (e.g., saying no, or avoiding potential perpetrators; fighting back); (3) encourage disclosure of any current or past abuse and differentiate between proper and improper types of secrets; and (4) convey the conviction that abuse is never a child's fault (Daro, 1994; Finkelhor & Dziuba-Leatherman, 1995; Wurtele, 1998).

However, there has been much debate in the literature about whether children should be expected to prevent their own abuse and whether these programs foster more guilt or blame by suggesting that the child should have stopped the abuse (Newman & Lutzker, 1990; Tharinger et al., 1988). Unfortunately, many of the available programs do not realistically address the dynamics of sexual abuse (including the less powerful, dependent nature of a child in relation to the known perpetrator). For example, expecting a young child to kick or run away from a would-be perpetrator (as suggested in some programs) has limited application to adult offender situations. Therefore, the presentation of self-protection strategies (e.g., saying no, escaping the situation) should be handled sensitively. Children in the audience may not have used these skills during a previous assault and may develop feelings of self-blame or guilt as a result of such instruction (Tharinger et al., 1988). Further, children who may later be victimized and "forget" to use such skills may feel an even greater sense of responsibility because they had been trained in how to avoid such an encounter. Some have argued that it is more realistic to expect children to learn to report, rather than actively struggle to prevent, their own abuse.

An additional concern is that, if this is the first exposure children have had to the topics of sex and sexuality, the experience might be quite negative, even scary. Thus, many (e.g., Tharinger et al., 1988) have called for the integration of sexual abuse prevention programs into broader curricula addressing a healthy awareness of one's body, as well as sex education. Another criticism is that these programs "may give parents and society a false sense of security" (Miller-Perrin & Perrin, 1999, p. 244). School-based programs should be just one part of a comprehensive and integrated prevention approach.

Program Effectiveness

Although there was a brief trend toward mass education in child abuse prevention, evaluation of the effectiveness of these programs was slow in developing. Some reasons for this may include (1) the uncertainty of program goals (i.e., some programs aim to increase children's knowledge of abuse while others focus on disclosures), (2) researchers often use self-designed measures with undetermined psychometric properties, (3) there is a lack of adequate sample sizes and control groups, and (4) control over other independent variables (such as cognitive development and emotional maturity) is difficult in school-based samples (Daro, 1994; Gentles & Cassidy, 1988).

Even with these limitations, more recent efforts to evaluate these programs have been undertaken, and some tentative conclusions may be drawn (for complete reviews, see Carroll, Miltenberger, & O'Neill, 1992; Daro, 1994; O'Donohue, Geer, & Elliott, 1992; Rispens et al., 1997; Wurtele, 1998). One might expect the primary question to be "Do prevention programs really *prevent* anything?" Unfortunately, this is a very difficult question to assess in that, more commonly, programs are evaluated in regard to evidence that students are acquiring and retaining knowledge, obtaining and employing skills, and disclosing ongoing or previous abuse.

Studies document that most programs using a variety of presentation styles (e.g., role-plays, discussions, films, modeling) do produce significant changes in children's knowledge of both sexual abuse and prevention skills (Daro, 1994; Finkelhor & Dziuba-Leatherman, 1995; Rispens et al., 1997; Sarno & Wurtele, 1997; Wurtele, 1998). Content areas typically covered include a continuum of touching, assertiveness skills, body ownership, and how to go about telling someone. Programs that were more comprehensive (i.e., covered a broader range of victimization experiences, identified a variety of possible perpetrators, involved parents, and allowed children a chance to practice skills) were shown to result in the greatest increase in sexual abuse knowledge, especially among those 10 to 11 years old (Finkelhor, Asdigian, & Dziuba-Leatherman, 1995). Studies regarding preschoolers' ability to learn prevention concepts have had varied results (Tutty, 1994; Sarno & Wurtele, 1997). Preschoolers more readily increase their knowledge of inappropriate touching but have greater difficulty learning to say no to adults and viewing perpetrators as adults (Tutty, 1994; Sarno & Wurtele, 1997). Those programs teaching a rule-based approach rather than a feeling-based approach were more helpful to younger children learning to discriminate between types of touching (Wurtele, 1998). Thus, most attempts to increase school-aged children's knowledge about child sexual abuse and about prevention skills are successful upon initial presentation, while the results with preschoolers are more varied.

While initial findings regarding knowledge acquisition are promising, only a limited number of studies have assessed the retention of this knowledge. Certainly, if the long-term effects of sexual abuse prevention programs are not tracked, there will be no evidence regarding the durability of the results (Carroll et al., 1992). The few studies that have followed up with children several weeks or months after a prevention program did find that children retained knowledge about sexual abuse and ways to prevent abuse from happening (Rispens et al., 1997). The combination of a film with another form of presentation (e.g., behavioral training, discussion, comic books, coloring books) may best serve to maintain these effects (Wurtele, Marrs, & Miller-Perrin, 1987).

While it is encouraging that children can learn and even retain abuse information, whether they develop and employ prevention skills is a different question. There has been comparatively little research conducted on the actual use of abuse prevention skills by children. Ethical issues make a true examination of the use of prevention skills by children in potentially abusive settings a challenge. Those implementing and studying prevention programs grounded in behavioral training with the use of modeling, role-plays, discussion, and social reinforcement do note that students are actively demonstrating the taught skills in that context. Direct instruction and opportunities for practice are particularly important, according to one metaanalysis (Rispens et al., 1997). While it is good to know that students can demonstrate the use of these skills at school, questions regarding generalization are, again, difficult to measure. Finkelhor and Dziuba-Leatherman (1995) did find that 42% of children who had practiced abuse prevention skills reported having used them at least once in a situation following the training. Self-reported rates such as these are encouraging but are somewhat unreliable, being influenced by social desirability and other related factors.

A few studies have attempted to investigate actual responses to potentially abusive situations. In one study, for example, children's responses to a "stranger" (actually, an investigator's confederate) who invited them to leave the school building was measured before and after the prevention program (Fryer, Krazier, Miyoshi, 1987). The results demonstrated that children could learn "stranger danger" type skills and even implement them. However, it should be noted that beyond the ethical questions in conducting this type of research, there are questions about the generalizability of the findings since most real-life abuse situations are with parents or persons previously familiar to the child as the perpetrators.

Wurtele and colleagues (1987) also reported that children who practiced their skills maintained their knowledge gains at a 3-month follow-up. However, follow-up scores are often lower than posttreatment scores, which would suggest that these programs should be repeated regularly, especially with younger and lower-SES students, to maintain their effectiveness (Finkelhor & Dziuba-Leatherman, 1995; Rispens et al., 1997).

In addition to increasing knowledge and enhancing skills, prevention programs may promote disclosure of previous or ongoing abuse. For some programs, this is an identified central goal, while for others disclosures are a positive side effect. In either case, most professionals agree that prevention programs do lead to disclosures. While postprogram disclosures are known to be common, specific findings in this area are rare and usually not published (Wurtele, 1998). Finkelhor and his colleagues (1995), however, found that, even after controlling for outside influences, children who received more comprehensive prevention programs disclosed higher levels of sexual abuse than those receiving less comprehensive exposure. Additionally, Hazzard and colleagues found that 1.5% of children disclosed ongoing sexual abuse and 3.8% reported past abuse within 6 weeks of receiving a three-session prevention program (Hazzard, Webb, Kleemeier, Angert, & Pohl, 1991). These results are encouraging, but future research should systematically evaluate this secondary outcome (Daro, 1994; Tharinger et al., 1988). This would mean that each study would have a control group for comparison and both pretraining and posttraining evaluations.

Even though empirical evidence in this area is lacking, those who have implemented programs consistently report high disclosure rates. Since it is not clear that they prevent anything, and it is clear that "prevention" programs do promote disclosures, some have argued that they could more appropriately be called "disclosure programs and . . . this is a more developmentally appropriate expectation" (Tharinger et al., 1988).

One additional aspect of program evaluation is the occurrence of unintended negative consequences. The issues of primary concern with prevention programs are the possible emotional (effects such as increased fear and anxiety) or behavioral effects (e.g., reluctance to engage in *any* physical contact with adults).

Studies examining anxiety through formal assessment measures have found no significant increases during or following the prevention programs (Wurtele, 1998). However, when researchers have asked children about their fears or worries related to possible abuse or adults in general, increased levels have been found (Finkelhor & Dziuba-Leatherman, 1995; Hazard et al., 1991). Parents of these children have also confirmed more anxiousness among children following the completion of these programs (Finkelhor & Dziuba-Leatherman, 1995). Interestingly, these authors also found that this reported worry by children and their parents was the greatest predictor in perceived program helpfulness. These "worried" children also reported employing the skills and concepts taught more often than those who reported not being worried at all. Two studies also revealed that children and their parents reported feeling more confident in the children's capacity to cope with potential abuse situations following participation in sexual abuse prevention programs (Binder & McNiel, 1987; Finkelhor & Dziuba-Leatherman, 1995). In light of these and other similar findings, some professionals have concluded that increased anxiety may be a reflection of effective efforts to convey important safety messages to children and may be an unavoidable cost of effective intervention (Garbarino, 1987).

School practitioners may conclude from these findings that there is no clear evidence that school-based sexual abuse prevention programs actually decrease victimization rates. Such a finding would be difficult to ever prove and has certainly not been empirically validated to date. However, there are positive secondary outcomes that support the ongoing provision of such programs. Therefore, school-based practitioners should consider the following conclusions drawn from the literature when deciding whether to offer a prevention program:

- ◆ Knowledge of signs and dangers is gained when information is presented age-appropriately.
- ◆ Younger children benefit from more visual material because of their limited abilities in retaining verbal presentations.
- ◆ Skills are developed when information is presented through multiple media (e.g., videos, storybooks or comic books, puppet shows, discussions) and when practice opportunities are provided.
- ◆ Comprehensive programs discussing both sexual abuse and other forms of victimization (e.g., physical abuse, bullying) are more effective.
- ◆ Repeated exposure enhances children's retention of concepts and skills.
- ◆ Programs involving parents are more effective than those not including parents.
- ◆ There is no conclusive evidence that instructor type (e.g., teacher, school psychologist, outside professional) during implementation makes a difference.
- ◆ There is some support for the fact that these programs provide a safe environment in which children may make disclosures.
- ◆ Increased levels of fear or anxiety may occur in some children but may not be reflective of a negative side effect so much as a reflection of greater receptivity or understanding of the information (Batchelor et al., 1990; Finkelhor & Dziuba-Leatherman, 1995; National Clearinghouse on Child Abuse and Neglect Information, 2000; Rispens et al., 1997; Tutty, 1994; Vevier & Tharinger, 1986).

If school practitioners and prevention planning teams decide to implement a personal safety program (see Table 7.3 for a list of guiding questions), they

TABLE 7.3. Guiding Questions for Prevention Program Selection

Content

◆ Does the curriculum teach assertiveness, build self-esteem, and help children develop problem-solving skills?
◆ Is it recommended and appropriate for the targeted age group?
◆ Does the curriculum portray a range of touches that are good and touches that are inappropriate?
◆ Does it describe verbal and physical abuse?
◆ Does it teach children to trust their own feelings and instincts?
◆ Does it teach children whom to tell if they are abused? Does it identify the range of people who make up a child's support system? Will the children understand that there are others they can tell if one person does not believe them?
◆ Do the pictures and examples avoid frightening children? If there are accompanying audiovisuals, do the pictures and music avoid frightening the children?
◆ Is the curriculum free from bias? Does the material include a variety of male and female, racial and ethnic, and urban and rural situations? Does it avoid stereotypes?
◆ Is the curriculum sensitive to the special learning needs of some children?
◆ Does the curriculum caution children about strangers without causing children to fear helpful strangers such as police officers? Are children made aware that most adults are trustworthy?
◆ Does the curriculum discuss family abuse in an appropriate way? Does it address adult, adolescent, and peer offenders?
◆ Is the curriculum compatible with the program's philosophy?
◆ Does the program stress behavioral enactment of personal safety skills and not simply discuss the issues?

Curriculum design features

◆ Is there a teacher's guide? Does it allow for the fact that the user might be uncomfortable teaching children about sexual abuse and may not be well informed on the subject?
◆ Are there supplemental materials, with instructions for use, for teachers and parents?
◆ Does it allow the user to pick and choose from a variety of appropriate activities?
◆ Does it help the user deal with disclosure if a child confides that he/she is a victim of maltreatment?
◆ Does it suggest ways to present the materials to parents and ways to involve them?
◆ Have the materials been pretested with the target population? What are the expected outcomes of using the curriculum? Are the stated purpose and outcome compatible?

Note. The material in this table was adapted from Koralek (1992).

should develop a plan to evaluate the program *and* make sure the findings are published or at least made known to the general public (Newman & Lutzker, 1990). More rigorous evaluations will continue to guide schools and communities in the approach they take to school-based prevention. However, simply teaching children to identify and resist sexual situations should not be the only approach in the prevention of child sexual abuse; activities involving parents should accompany these programs.

Secondary Prevention

In addition to their many roles in primary prevention, school practitioners can be involved in secondary prevention, responding to those most at risk. At this level, school practitioners may also develop and implement parent education programs but with specific subgroups. For example, programs supporting adolescent mothers may involve parenting classes, support groups, or in-school day cares. School practitioners can play an instrumental role in educating school administrators about the long-term benefits of supporting these students with school resources. Additionally, parent education programs within the school and community that are targeting at-risk families may place greater emphasis on parental stress, parent psychological functioning, and interpersonal relationships, especially those with high levels of conflict.

Tertiary Prevention

The third level of prevention includes services targeted at known victims and perpetrators of child maltreatment. At this level of prevention in the schools, practitioners are primarily working with children and educators following the identification or reporting of child maltreatment. These direct and indirect roles have been detailed earlier in this volume.

Support

There are many ways practitioners may indirectly be involved in tertiary prevention such as consultative efforts that provide information and, more importantly, emotional support to school personnel and parents (James & Burch, 1999) (see Chapters 3 and 6 for more details). For example, school practitioners may provide staff with information or forms useful in documenting observations or disclosures of maltreatment, or more broadly serve as role models for both educators and parents to illustrate how both parties can work together effectively. Home–school collaboration may increase at this level of prevention to encourage an open dialogue between both environments in which the child may demonstrate progress or setbacks.

Coordination

Once a child has been identified as maltreated and a report has been made, school mental health providers may establish themselves in the role of coordinator (see Chapter 4 for more information). Children who have been maltreated will likely receive a variety of services, with some of these taking place in-house and others occurring in the community. Thus, it is important that someone, preferably a school-based practitioner, coordinate these efforts to ensure that services are being received and the child's needs are being met, and to avoid duplication of services. This role may be easier if the practitioner has already established professional links with local mental health providers and CPS workers. Additionally, it is important to have one contact person within the school system through whom information about progress and interventions may be conveyed. School mental health providers could best serve this role, as they have more training and experience with both educational and psychological issues.

Direct Service Provider

Finally, school-based practitioners may choose to provide treatment to children and/or their families. This is a role that should be chosen only by those who are competent in the treatment of child abuse and neglect and who are willing and can devote substantial time to this type of service (see Chapter 5 for a more in-depth review). In addition to individual or family therapy, which would typically address the issue of maltreatment, school-based practitioners may feel more competent and willing to provide support and ancillary treatment. Ancillary treatment might include working with children in small topic-based groups (e.g., divorce, peer relations, anger management) or coordinating parent support groups to be held at the school (e.g., Parents Anonymous, Alcoholics Anonymous).

CONCLUSION

Child maltreatment is a complex multifaceted problem that demands a complex multifaceted solution. If schools do not engage in the prevention process, then they become part of the problem (Mayhall & Norgard, 1983). It is not enough, however, to just provide programs teaching children how to recognize and respond to abusive situations. School-based practitioners have the training and expertise to take a broader role in primary, secondary, and tertiary prevention efforts on-site and in the community. They can also use their knowledge and position within the schools to encourage administrators and school boards to make better use of their unique resources, whether it be staff diversity, location, and/or superior facilities.

The majority of schools have provided, and will continue to provide, personal safety and victimization prevention programs. These reflect a highly cost-effective approach, reaching nearly all American children with information about the various types of child maltreatment. Although not all children attending these programs will be personally affected by child maltreatment, the information given them will serve to educate future teachers, doctors, psychologists, and police officers who will most likely have to confront potential child abuse and neglect in their occupational roles daily (Sudermann et al., 1995). When asked to develop and/or implement a victimization prevention program, school-based practitioners should be aware of the strengths, limitations, and unintended consequences associated with each. Programs that are developmentally sensitive, involve parents, and are presented through a variety of media (e.g., role-plays, storybooks, videos) seem to produce the most positive responses from students, parents, and school personnel (Daro, 1994; Finkelhor & Dziuba-Leatherman, 1995; Wurtele, 1998).

Regardless of which level of prevention and which type of program is selected, school personnel will continue to play a key role in child maltreatment prevention. This only seems fitting since protecting and enhancing the lives of children is every educator's responsibility.

CHAPTER 8

◆◆◆

Self-Care: Identifying and Preventing Compassion Fatigue

◆

with SARAH E. STEINKAMP

This volume provides evidence that it is critical for school personnel to be involved in the response to child maltreatment. Child abuse is occurring at alarming rates; the effects are potentially devastating; and the unmet needs are many. So, in theory, school personnel should be eager to respond in the various roles described earlier, that is, identifying, reporting, and intervening. In reality, however, if they are honest, many school personnel would admit that they are not so eager to get involved. It is frankly easier to not notice fairly obvious signs, conclude that there is not quite enough reason to suspect in order to make a report, and to make rigid policies about what is beyond the scope of school-based practice. Why is it easier not to get involved? First, much of the school professional population is tired, stressed, and burned out. For example, 40% of school psychologists experience significant symptoms of burnout (Huebner, 1992; Mills & Huebner, 1998). One study even reported that 35% of school psychologists were considering leaving the profession (Huebner, 1993). Such factors as the large ratio of students to psychologists, the lack of social support, isolation, and inadequate resources make the job nearly unbearable for many (Huebner, 1994; Mills & Huebner, 1998). Meeting federal mandates regarding special education eligibility, as an example, is incredibly demanding itself for many school mental health professionals. Yet, this primary duty for school psychologists can also lead to job dissatisfaction, as some may wish their roles could be expanded. Regardless of their assign-

Sarah E. Steinkamp, MS, is a doctoral student in the School Psychology Program at Illinois State University, Normal, Illinois.

ments, many school professionals feel they do not have the time and energy for many other important issues . . . and there are many.

Certainly child maltreatment is a compelling issue, but this is not the only pressing concern schools must face. Beyond the academic basics and eligibility concerns, schools are faced with multiple other mental health and societal issues. In the wake of numerous shootings that occurred throughout the country, school violence has remained in the forefront of many communities' concerns. An increasingly diverse student population demands special sensitivities and accommodations, and in some locales, racial tensions remain a concern. Many students are depressed, some are addicted to alcohol or drugs, and others are dealing with family changes, and the list could go on and on.

So there are many legitimate reasons to not want to get involved in child maltreatment, as there are already more than enough serious concerns to address. But perhaps, again, if school professionals are totally honest, their avoiding, not noticing, and not getting involved in child maltreatment issues is partially attributable to the emotional toll it exacts. It is disturbing to really consider how many children in one's class might be victims of abuse or neglect. It is upsetting to consider that the girl sitting alone in the cafeteria might not simply be "shy" but also be filled with self-loathing because of some abusive relationship in her family. It is easier to suggest that parents look into Ritalin for ADHD than to seriously consider whether the child's agitation may be due to abuse he/she is experiencing rather than a neurological problem. And yet, discovering maltreatment or hearing children's disclosures of physical and emotional hurt can be the most painful experience of all. Although being involved is critical to a child's safety and recovery, it may come at a steep cost to those in the helping role (e.g., teachers, social workers, school psychologists, nurses).

Persons involved in child maltreatment and similar fields have acknowledged the emotional energy it takes to get involved. There is recognition of the "cost of caring" (Figley, 1989). Interchangeable concepts such as compassion fatigue, vicarious traumatization, the ripple effect, and secondary traumatic stress (STS) describe the phenomenon that may result from working with suffering children (Figley & Kleber, 1995).

DEFINITIONS

Compassion fatigue is "the natural, predictable, treatable, and preventable unwanted consequence of working with suffering people" (Figley, 1995b, p. 4). It is viewed by some as an occupational hazard that results from empathizing and identifying with a traumatized person or child to the point that there are "changes in the self that parallel those experienced by trauma survivors themselves" (Pearlman, 1995, p. 52). Similarly, secondary traumatic stress consists of behaviors and emotions that are a "consequence of caring between two people, one of whom has been initially traumatized and the other of whom is affected by the first's traumatic experiences" (Figley & Kleber, 1995, p. 92). The symptoms of stress that result are said to be secondary because they are not a direct response to a traumatic event but rather an indirect response based on contact with the victim. Compassion fatigue does not reflect pathology in the helper, nor does the traumatized individual deliberately produce it (Pearlman & Mac Ian, 1995).

As alluded to previously and further supported by Pearlman's (1995) statement, "anyone who engages empathically with trauma survivors is vulnerable" (p. 52). No one is immune to the disturbing thoughts, feelings, and details of children's maltreatment. In fact, emergency workers report it is *children's* trauma that they find most disturbing of all the trauma they encounter (Figley, 1995a). Thus, school practitioners who may face the direct or indirect discovery and disclosure of children's maltreatment repeatedly over time are most likely to develop compassion fatigue. Although there is increasingly more literature in this area, there has been no direct mention of compassion fatigue's applicability to school mental health professionals.

BACKGROUND AND HISTORY OF THE FIELD

The indirect effects that mental health professionals experience as a result of working with trauma survivors has only been recognized during the past decade. One contributing factor to the recent recognition is the increased awareness of the large number of traumatic events that occur in the lives of children and families and the impact that traumatic events have on so many people "beyond the victim" (Figley, 1995b; Figley & Kleber, 1995). A second factor has been the inclusion of the mental health diagnosis posttraumatic stress disorder (PTSD) in the third edition of the American Psychiatric Association's (APA) *Diagnostic and Statistical Manual of Mental Disorders* (DSM-III; American Psychiatric Association, 1980).

PTSD is a diagnosis that incorporates symptoms that have been observed and recorded among traumatized persons. Over the past twenty years, the accumulation of empirical research has helped to validate the disorder, and the research literature has grown tremendously. Most of the research, however, has focused only on people who were directly "in harm's way" and excluded those who provided care to them and were traumatized in the process (i.e., some mental health professionals, counselors, school psychologists) (Figley, 1995b; Figley & Kleber, 1995). Some have even declared that PTSD should really stand for *primary* traumatic stress disorder rather than posttraumatic stress disorder (Figley, 1995a). Subsequent revisions of the DSM-III (i.e., DSM-III-R and DSM-IV) have modified the symptom criteria over the years, and the DSM-IV indicates that the *witnessing* of another's trauma or *knowledge of* another person's traumatic experience can be traumatizing, even without actually being harmed or threatened with harm yourself (American Psychiatric Association, 1994). From this, researchers (e.g., Figley, 1995a, 1995b; Pearlman & Mac Ian, 1995) believe that therapists, counselors, and other professionals who work with trauma victims are at risk of experiencing symptoms of PTSD or compassion fatigue. School practitioners should also remember that the families of the traumatized children they work with may also be indirectly affected. Thus, helping them to understand their experience and find resources to assist in coping may be a much-needed component in resolving the family's problems in the long run.

IDENTIFICATION

Although compassion fatigue typically emerges suddenly without much warning, the symptoms may not be understood as problematic by school-based practitioners, as they are often misinterpreted as "caring" (Figley, 1995b). Initial effects may be manifested in feelings of helplessness and confusion, as the practitioner is confronted with a sense of powerlessness and a disruption to one's current beliefs, or worldview (Figley & Kleber, 1995). Ongoing symptoms are nearly identical to the PTSD symptoms experienced by survivors (Figley, 1995b; Figley & Kleber, 1995). The following are characteristics of compassion fatigue that school-based practitioners may notice in themselves.

1. *Cannot stop thinking about abused children.* While our aim in this volume is to encourage school professionals to consider child abuse issues, becoming overwhelmed by these thoughts is not helpful to anyone. Practitioners may feel they cannot get the issue of child maltreatment off their mind, or thoughts or images that may be distressing may just suddenly "pop up."

2. *Dreams/nightmares.* Practitioners may begin to have recurrent dreams or nightmares, sometimes specifically involving the children or families they are concerned most about and at other times involving the more general themes of abuse, violence, or trying to escape from harm.

3. *Flashbacks or dissociation.* Children's maltreatment may trigger for some practitioners thoughts and feelings of (sometimes similar) traumatic events in their own lives. Therefore, they may begin reexperiencing their own trauma through flashbacks or dissociative episodes.

4. *Negative health consequences.* Sleeping problems, depression, psychosomatic illnesses, eating disorders, and increased use of drugs or alcohol are of-

ten reported by professionals experiencing compassion fatigue (Figley & Kleber, 1995; Herman, 1992; Ryan & Lane, 1997b).

5. *No longer feel safe.* "Repeated exposure to stories of human rapacity and cruelty inevitably challenges the therapist's basic faith and heightens her sense of personal vulnerability" (Herman, 1992, p. 141). The practitioner may become hypervigilant, expecting violence at every turn, and begin to doubt the safety and certainty once felt about people and the world.

6. *Relationships are negatively affected.* As beliefs about the world being a safe place are challenged, school professionals may become more distrustful of others, even those close to them. This may be evidenced through a developed paranoia regarding their children's care (i.e., suspicious of everyone involved in their care) or difficulty with intimacy with their partner.

7. *Clinical judgment becomes skewed.* School-based practitioners may begin to see child abuse under every rock. There are many legitimate cases of ADHD that have nothing to do with child abuse. Not every child with nightmares is abused; some children are simply anxious.

8. *Work performance is affected.* In response to their emotional reactions to children's maltreatment, some practitioners may try to avoid their intense thoughts and feelings by becoming more involved at work, while others may begin to call in sick or miss work more often (Figley & Kleber, 1995). Additionally, these professionals may begin to doubt their own competency and have a sense of helplessness or guilt. They may believe that they are not "making a difference," being continually faced with more children who have been maltreated. They may experience "witness guilt," which leads them to overextend their roles and risk burnout in their jobs (Herman, 1992).

9. *Withdrawal.* As school professionals come to experience many of these symptoms, they may feel as though something is wrong with them or that others are not affected in the same way they are. Therefore, they may begin to isolate themselves from coworkers and even family and friends (Ryan & Lane, 1997b).

10. *Emotional exhaustion.* School personnel have many roles and responsibilities that may deplete their energy even without working with traumatized children. Emotional exhaustion is also a common symptom of the parallel, but different, concept of burnout (Figley, 1995b).

In addition to these symptoms that are similar to the diagnostic criteria of PTSD, professionals working with trauma victims may also experience a number of other changes within themselves. Pearlman (1995) has observed that secondary exposure to traumatic events can radically affect your sense of self or identity (e.g., woman, helper, mother), your worldview (e.g., moral principles), your spirituality (e.g., hope, meaning in life), and your sensitivity and affect tolerance (i.e., you may lose touch with your feelings).

To better understand the impact of compassion fatigue, consider, for example, the following scenario. Ms. Sims is an elementary school counselor in a school district that has provided prevention programming on sexual abuse as part of the curriculum for the past three years. After a lesson focusing on the importance of telling a trusted person if sexual abuse occurs, a 9-year-old student, Caitlin, approaches Ms. Sims. Caitlin discloses to Ms. Sims that her father has been sexually abusing her for as long as she can remember; she even goes on to share the graphic details of her father sexually violating her on several occasions. Caitlin's disclosure, as it turns out, was but one of many traumatic stories that children revealed to Ms. Sims in the wake of the abuse curriculum. As an apparent consequence, Ms. Sims began to exhibit a number of symptoms of compassion fatigue. For example, Ms. Sims became unable to sleep at night. When finally she was able to doze off, she would often awaken from nightmares about Caitlin and Caitlin's father. Ms. Sims also began to avoid interactions and conversations with many of the children who had disclosed. When speaking to them, she noticed that she would often readily recall the exact date of their disclosures and the details that each had shared. Finally, Ms. Sims began calling in sick to work several days a month. She has since been experiencing severe headaches and stomach upset. Although Ms. Sims does not exhibit all of the possible symptoms of compassion fatigue, it is evident that she has been indirectly traumatized as a result of her work.

School psychologists, social workers, counselors, teachers, and other school personnel all have contact with a large number of children and will encounter more than one child who has been a victim of abuse or neglect or some other traumatic event. It is, therefore, likely that these school personnel will encounter compassion fatigue at some point during their career. Table 8.1 provides an extensive list of possible signs, or "red flags," to watch for if you have ongoing contact with children who are victims of child maltreatment.

Identifying warning signs and symptoms of compassion fatigue is crucial to the health and well-being of individuals working with victims of trauma. Additionally, self-care is a preventative step from further unintentionally harming trauma victims. As stated by Saakvitne and Pearlman (1996), "it is easier to protect yourself . . . if you know your vulnerabilities" (p. 51). When symptoms are overlooked and unattended to by school practitioners, "this secondary exposure to trauma may cause helpers to inflict additional pain on the originally traumatized" (Figley, 1995b, p. 4). Practitioners, who may unknowingly begin to withdraw from traumatized clients, minimize the clients' stories, or provide a less-than-sensitive response (as a result of their own difficulty coping with the traumatic material) are certainly not functioning in the best interests of the student. Thus, an important first step to self-care is being able to identify and recognize the signs and symptoms of compassion fatigue or secondary traumatic stress. Additionally, it is important to learn what factors make some professionals more vulnerable to compassion fatigue than

TABLE 8.1. Warning Signs of Compassion Fatigue

1. Overwhelming feelings (e.g., feelings of severe anger and rage toward the perpetrator)
2. Feeling that others cannot and are not to be trusted and/or changes in self-trust
3. Feelings of helplessness for self and the victim (e.g., sense of giving up)
4. An inability to separate work from personal life
5. Feelings of sadness and depression
6. An inability to engage in social activities and leisure activities previously enjoyed
7. Finding yourself questioning your religion and/or spirituality
8. An increase in the consumption of alcohol or other substances
9. Increased illness or problems with health
10. Withdrawal from family and friends
11. Increased tension and stress in your life
12. An increase in the amount of work hours
13. An inability to get the victim or victims out of your mind
14. Feelings of wanting to "rescue" the victim
15. Recognition of identifying with the victim (e.g., noticing similarities in the victims' experience and your own experiences)
16. Feeling that no one could possibly understand what you are going through
17. Questioning your worldview and your beliefs about the meaning of life
18. Avoidance of specific cues that represent aspects of the traumatic incidents (e.g., traumatized children themselves, or movies or books with trauma-related themes)
19. Feelings of a foreshortened future
20. Problems in your interpersonal relationships (e.g., marital discord)
21. Hypersensitivity to your own and/or your children's safety (or other children in your family)
22. Suspiciousness of everyone as a possible abuser of children
23. Increase in professional errors (e.g., boundaries, setting limits)
24. Loss of hope
25. Loss of or changes in self-esteem
26. Doubting competencies
27. Ineffective coping
28. Feelings of cynicism and pessimism
29. Feelings of resentment
30. Symptoms that parallel PTSD diagnostic criteria

Note. Information for this table was obtained from the following sources: Figley (1995a, 1995b); Herman (1992); Pearlman (1995); Pearlman and Mac Ian (1995); and Ryan and Lane (1997b).

others. Authors and researchers have discussed a number of factors that may contribute to a greater risk of compassion fatigue (e.g., Beaton & Murphy, 1995; Saakvitne & Pearlman, 1996).

CONTRIBUTING FACTORS

Current clinical and empirical investigation suggests several reasons for the development of compassion fatigue among psychologists or therapists. The most fundamental factor contributing to compassion fatigue is empathy (Figley, 1995a). The ability to identify with and understand a victim's traumatic experience is necessary for effective treatment, but it may be painful to hear, incomprehensible, or overwhelming for the school-based practitioner (Ryan & Lane, 1997b). Hearing the details of a child's brutal beating or invasive sexual molestation may come as a harsh shock to those close to the child. It is thought that the most effective therapists (i.e., those who have a greater capacity for empathy) are at the highest risk for compassion fatigue (Figley, 1995b); so it is the very aspect that makes them best able to help a child reveal his/her innermost thoughts and feelings that also places the helper at the greatest risk of harm.

Additionally, many of the individuals who are helping others work through their trauma have themselves personally experienced some type of traumatic event (Figley, 1995a). For example, 26% of female psychologists in one study reported a history of child sexual abuse (Schauben & Frazier, 1995), while nearly 60% of outpatient therapists in another study had experienced physical, emotional, or sexual abuse as a child or adult (Kassam-Adams, 1995). For interventionists who have their own history of child maltreatment, issues of vicarious trauma are even more salient. At one level these individuals may have unique gifts and abilities in responding to child abuse issues (i.e., they may be better at noticing signs of abuse or neglect or may have a more genuine empathic response), but for some survivors listening to a child's trauma may trigger a host of unwanted feelings and memories. Thus, especially if their trauma is unresolved, this may heighten their level of distress. However, limited empirical findings are inconclusive about whether a clinician's personal history of trauma is a risk factor for compassion fatigue (Kassam-Adams, 1995; Pearlman & Mac Ian, 1995; Schauben & Frazier, 1995). Some have found that it is more a function of the number of trauma cases on one's caseload.

Exposure to traumatized individuals has also been indicated as a possible risk factor (Figley, 1995a; Schauben & Frazier, 1995). The more maltreated children one comes into contact with, the greater the likelihood one's beliefs may be challenged and one's sense of control over life may be altered. The number of cases involving child maltreatment school professionals are working with should be closely monitored as well as related activities that might increase their exposure to such material. Additionally, one's attitude toward the helping process, which may also be directly related to the number of maltreatment cases one works with, should be evaluated. It has been noted that those who are most vulnerable to compassion fatigue are those who "view themselves as saviors or at least as rescuers" (Figley, 1989, pp. 144–145).

Newer and inexperienced mental health professionals appear to be at greater risk for developing compassion fatigue (Pearlman & Mac Ian, 1995). Not only may these professionals be new to their particular field (e.g., school psychology), but they may also have limited training and experience in working with maltreated children. It is also highly likely that they have not been sufficiently warned about how compassion fatigue is such a natural by-product of working with these children. Reported stress levels for newer professionals are greatest for those with a personal history of trauma (Pearlman & Mac Ian, 1995).

Finally, sufficient support from colleagues and supervisors is a fundamental requirement in counteracting negative effects from working with maltreated children. "Just as no survivor can recover alone, no therapist can work with trauma alone" (Herman, 1992, p. 141). To combat the negative impact of another's traumatic experience, school practitioners must ensure opportunities to express their emotional reactions as well as gain help and support in what to do. One must find a "safe, structured, and regular forum for reviewing" these cases. For example, individual supervision or peer support groups could be requested from others in one's setting or field. Professional support will aid practitioners in understanding that they are not alone and in normalizing their reactions.

Additional risk factors may include demographic variables (e.g., age, ethnicity), personality characteristics (e.g., sense of humor or lack thereof), individual history of psychiatric symptoms (e.g., acute symptomology of PTSD), and the nature of the helper (e.g., what additional life stressors are already present) (Beaton & Murphy, 1995; Saakvitne & Pearlman, 1996). Readers interested in a personal assessment of one's risk for compassion fatigue are referred to Saakvitne and Pearlman (1996). In their book, worksheets are provided to help further identify signs and symptoms as well as the contributing factors cited earlier.

PREVENTION AND INTERVENTION

Knowing what the signs and contributing factors of compassion fatigue are, what can school professionals do to keep emotionally healthy enough to stay involved and concerned about child maltreatment? In a general statement Pearlman (1995) captures the answer by stating that you should do the "self-nuturing, self-building things" you would have your clients do. Some specific examples of this follow.

1. *Try to keep a balanced caseload.* There are pros and cons of having a "district expert" on child maltreatment issues. On the one hand, this person can be hired to consult or provide training on this topic. This person can keep up with the field and provide a valuable resource to others in the district. If one person, however, is assigned the majority of child abuse cases to deal with, the emotional drain on that person may be too great.

2. *Ongoing supervision.* If someone is a new professional or new to the sub-

ject of child abuse, the need for supervision, hopefully, is clearly recognized. However, perhaps not as obvious is the need for peer supervision for even the most seasoned professional. Beyond simply the "Do I call this one in?" or "To whom should I refer this child?" clinicians need the opportunity to process their involvement in these difficult cases. What was it like to have the child tell you that he wished he never told you because now he is in bigger trouble? How did it feel to have this child disclose such horrific abuse? How does this remind you of your own childhood? These are questions that might give anyone cause for reflection and require support from others.

3. *Continued education and training.* Just as with supervision, both novice and veteran school professionals should continue to learn more about child maltreatment and the various roles they may play in detection, intervention, and prevention.

4. *Thought-stopping techniques.* Professionals may need to make a conscious effort to "turn off" intrusive or obsessive thoughts. For example, one might say aloud, "I have done all I can, I am not going to think about it tonight."

5. *Keep life in balance.* Becoming obsessed with the issue is not helpful. Those who can view work as only one aspect of who they are and what their purpose is are less apt to burn out or rest their self-concept and self-worth on it.

6. *Peaceful pursuits, hobbies, creative endeavors.* School professionals may find peace and comfort by paying attention to their own spiritual lives. Hobbies or interests (e.g., writing, gardening, playing music, painting) unrelated to child maltreatment or any aspect of work may help to cushion one against the negative effects of trauma work.

7. *Enjoy healthy relationships.* In order to maintain a personal connection with others, school practitioners should spend sufficient time with family and friends. Communities of faith may be an important resource. Additionally, school practitioners should try to work with "nonclinical age-mates of their client population in order to maintain a sense of normality" (Ryan & Lane, 1997b, p. 472).

8. *Take care of your body.* Typical suggestions for general stress reduction also apply for those working with maltreated children. Eating healthy and having an exercise plan, along with relaxation exercises, are common coping methods.

9. *Set boundaries between home and work.* Practitioners should avoid playing therapist to family and friends. Some even caution against socializing with coworkers if work cannot be left at school. Practitioners should "give themselves permission to leave work behind" (Ryan & Lane, 1997b, p. 473).

10. *Address psychological concerns.* Certainly, one should seek psychological help if he/she is experiencing compassion fatigue symptoms and/or has an unresolved history of trauma (Dutton & Rubinstein, 1995).

A final area of prevention rests with training programs. Trainers should directly address the issue of compassion fatigue. Munroe (1995) argues that professionals must be taught not only the indicators and risk factors of abuse but also how to cope with their exposure to traumatized individuals.

CONCLUSION

School professionals are often faced with many serious concerns in their work with children and adolescents, but often they do not have the time, flexibility, or resources to address them all. One area on which many school-based practitioners are increasingly choosing to direct their focus is child maltreatment. Although "the reward of engagement is the sense of an enriched life" (Herman, 1992, p. 153), many practitioners may pay the cost of caring along the way. Figley (1995b) concludes two main points regarding working with traumatized individuals: "(a) do not do this work alone and (b) monitor your responses to the work through your own careful attendance to your process and through supervision by your trusted colleagues" (p. xv). Children need school professionals to stay involved and concerned about the problem of child maltreatment. Thus, increased awareness of compassion fatigue and effective implementation of self-care techniques are important for all concerned.

◆◆◆
References
◆

Abrahams, N., Casey, K., & Daro, D. (1992). Teachers' knowledge, attitudes, and beliefs about child abuse and its prevention. *Child Abuse and Neglect, 16,* 229–238.

Adelman, H. S., & Taylor, L. (1998a). Addressing barriers to learning: Beyond school-linked services and full-service schools. *American Journal of Orthopsychiatry, 67,* 408–421.

Adelman, H. S., & Taylor, L. (1998b). Reframing mental health in schools and expanding school reform. *Educational Psychologist, 33,* 135–152.

Alexander, P. C. (1992). Application of attachment theory to the study of sexual abuse. *Journal of Consulting and Clinical Psychology, 60,* 185–195.

Allen, C. (1991). *Women and men who sexually abuse children: A comparative study.* Orwell, VT: Safer Society Press.

American Association for Protecting Children. (1985). *Highlights of official child neglect and abuse reporting,* 1983. Denver, CO: American Humane Association.

American Association for Protecting Children. (1988). *Highlights of official child neglect and abuse reporting,* 1986. Denver, CO: American Humane Association.

American Psychiatric Association. (1980). *Diagnostic and statistical manual of mental disorders* (3rd ed.). Washington, DC: Author.

American Psychiatric Association. (1994). *Diagnostic and statistical manual of mental disorders* (4th ed.). Washington, DC: Author.

Anderson, E. M., & Levine, M. (1999). Concerns about allegations of child sexual abuse against teachers and the teaching environment. *Child Abuse and Neglect, 23,* 833–843.

Araji, S. K. (1997). *Sexually aggressive children: Coming to understand them.* Thousand Oaks, CA: Sage.

Arata, C. M. (1998). To tell or not to tell: Current functioning of child sexual abuse survivors who disclosed their victimization. *Child Maltreatment, 3,* 63–71.

Bandura, A. (1977). *Social learning theory.* Englewood Cliffs, NJ: Prentice-Hall.

Batchelor, E. S., Dean, R. S., Gridley, B., & Batchelor, B. (1990). Reports of child sexual abuse in the schools. *Psychology in the Schools, 27,* 131–137.

179

Bates, R. P. (1980). Child abuse and neglect: A medical priority. In R. Volpe, M. Breton, & J. Mitton (Eds.), *The maltreatment of the school-aged child* (pp. 45–58). Lexington, MA: Lexington Books.

Beaton, R. D., & Murphy, S. A. (1995). Working with people in crisis: Research implications. In C. R. Figley (Ed.), *Compassion fatigue: Coping with secondary traumatic stress disorder in those who treat the traumatized* (pp. 51–81). New York: Brunner/Mazel.

Beitchman, J. H., Zucker, K. J., Hood, J. E., DaCosta, G. A., & Akman, D. (1991). A review of the short-term effects of child sexual abuse. *Child Abuse and Neglect, 15,* 537–556.

Bergner, R. M. (1990). Father–daughter incest: Degradation and recovery from degradation. *Advances in Descriptive Psychology, 5,* 285–305.

Berliner, L., & Rawlings, L. (1991). *A treatment manual: Children with sexual behavior problems.* Unpublished manuscript, Harborview Sexual Assault Center, University of Washington, Seattle, WA.

Bernstein, S. (1997). *A family that fights.* Morton Grove, IL: Albert Whitman.

Binder, R. L., & McNiel, D. E. (1987). Evaluation of a school-based sexual abuse prevention program: Cognitive and emotional effects. *Child Abuse and Neglect, 11,* 497–506.

Black, M. M., & Dubowitz, H. (1999). Child neglect: Research recommendations and future directions. In H. Dubowitz (Ed.), *Neglected children: Research, practice, and policy* (pp. 261–277). Thousand Oaks, CA: Sage.

Bloomquist, M. L. (1996). *Skills training for children with behavior disorders: A parent and therapist guidebook.* New York: Guilford Press.

Bowlby, J. (1982). *Attachment and loss: Vol. 1. Attachment.* New York: Basic Books.

Brassard, M. R., & Gelardo, M. S. (1987). Psychological maltreatment: The unifying construct in child abuse and neglect. *School Psychology Review, 16,* 127–136.

Brassard, M. R., Tyler, A., & Kehle, T. J. (1983). Sexually abused children: Identification and suggestions for intervention. *School Psychology Review, 12,* 93–96.

Briere, J. N. (1992). *Child abuse trauma: Theory and treatment of the lasting effects.* Newbury Park, CA: Sage.

Briere, J. N., & Conte, J. R. (1993). Self-reported amnesia for abuse in adults molested as children. *Journal of Traumatic Stress, 6,* 21–31.

Briere, J. N., & Elliott, D. M. (1994). Immediate and long-term impacts of child sexual abuse. In R. E. Behrman (Ed.), *The future of children: Sexual abuse of children* (pp. 54–69). Los Altos, CA: The Center for the Future of Children, The David and Lucile Packard Foundation.

Broadhurst, D. D. (1980). The effect of child abuse and neglect on the school-aged child. In R. Volpe, M. Breton, & J. Mitton (Eds.), *The maltreatment of the school-aged child* (pp. 19–26). Lexington, MA: Lexington Books.

Bromfield, R., Bromfield, D., & Weiss, B. (1988). Influence of the sexually abused label on perceptions of a child's failure. *Journal of Educational Research, 82,* 96–98.

Browne, A., & Finkelhor, D. (1986). Impact of child sexual abuse: A review of the research. *Psychological Bulletin, 99,* 66–77.

Burgess, A. W., & Groth, N. (1980). Sexual victimization of children. In R. Volpe, M. Breton, & J. Mitton (Eds.), *The maltreatment of the school-aged child* (pp. 79–90). Lexington, MA: Lexington Books.

Burton, J. E., & Rasmussen, L. A. (1998). *Treating children with sexually abusive behavior problems: Guidelines for child and parent intervention.* New York: Haworth Maltreatment and Trauma Press.

Cantwell, H. B. (1980). Child neglect. In C. H. Kempe & R. E. Helfer (Eds.), *The battered child* (pp. 183–197). Chicago: University of Chicago Press.

Caplan, G. (1995). Types of mental health consultation. *Journal of Educational and Psychological Consultation, 6,* 7–21.

Carlson, B. E. (1984). Children's observations of interparental violence. In A. R. Roberts (Ed.), *Battered women and their families: Intervention strategies and treatment programs* (pp. 147–157). New York: Springer.

Carlson, V., Cicchetti, D., Barnett, D., & Braunwald, K. (1989). Disorganized/disoriented attachment relationships in maltreated infants. *Developmental Psychology, 25,* 525–531.

Carroll, L. A., Miltenberger, R. G., & O' Neill, H. K. (1992). A review and critique of research evaluating child sexual abuse prevention programs. *Education and Treatment of Children, 15,* 335–354.

Center for Mental Health in Schools. (1997). *School-based client consultation, referral, and management of care.* Los Angeles: School Mental Health Project, Department of Psychology, University of California–Los Angeles.

Cheston, S. E. (1991). *Making effective referrals: The therapeutic process.* New York: Gardner Press.

Christenson, S. L. (1995). Supporting home–school collaboration. In A. Thomas & T. Grimes (Eds.), *Best practices in school psychology—III* (pp. 253–269). Washington, DC: National Association of School Psychologists.

Cohen, J. A., & Mannarino, A. P. (1993). A treatment model for sexually abused preschoolers. *Journal of Interpersonal Violence, 8,* 115–131.

Conti, A. P. (1975). Variables related to contacting/not contacting counseling services recommended by school psychologists. *Journal of School Psychology, 13,* 41–50.

Corder, B. F., Haizlip, T., & DeBoer, P. (1990). A pilot study for a structured, time-limited therapy group for sexually abused pre-adolescent children. *Child Abuse and Neglect, 14,* 243–251.

Cosentino, C. E. (1989). Child sexual abuse prevention: Guidelines for the school psychologist. *School Psychology Review, 18,* 371–385.

Courtois, C. A. (1993). *Adult survivors of child sexual abuse.* Milwaukee: Families International.

Crenshaw, W. B., Crenshaw, L. M., & Lichtenberg, J. W. (1995). When educators confront child abuse: An analysis of the decision to report. *Child Abuse and Neglect, 19,* 1095–1113.

Crick, N. R., & Dodge, K. A. (1996). Social information-processing mechanisms on reactive and proactive aggression. *Child Development, 67,* 993–1002.

Crisci, G., Lay, M., & Lowenstein, L. (1998). *Paper dolls and paper airplanes: Therapeutic exercises for sexually traumatized children.* Indianapolis, IN: Kidsrights.

Cruise, T. K. (1999). An examination of differences between peer- vs. adult-perpetrated child sexual abuse: The effects and mediators (Doctoral dissertation, Illinois State University, 1998). *Dissertation Abstracts International, 60*(04), b1847.

Cummings, E. M., & Davies, P. (1994). *Children and marital conflict: The impact of family dispute and resolution.* New York: Guilford Press.

Cunningham, C., & MacFarlane, K. (1996). *When children abuse: Group treatment strategies for children with impulse control problems.* Brandon, VT: Safer Society Press.

Daro, D. A. (1994). Prevention of child sexual abuse. In R. E. Behrman (Ed.), *The future of children: Sexual abuse of children* (pp. 198–223). Los Altos, CA: The Center for the Future of Children, The David and Lucile Packard Foundation.

Davis, W. W. (1997, August). *Implementing effective school-linked school-based mental health programs.* Paper presented at the 105th Annual Convention of the American Psychological Association, Chicago, IL.

Deblinger, E., & Heflin, A. H. (1996). *Treatment for sexually abused children and their nonoffending parents: A cognitive-behavioral approach.* Thousand Oaks, CA: Sage.

Deblinger, E., McLeer, S. V., & Henry, D. (1990). Cognitive behavioral treatment for sexually abused children suffering post-traumatic stress: Preliminary findings. *Journal of the American Academy of Child and Adolescent Psychiatry, 29,* 747–752.

Deisz, R., Doueck, H. J., George, N., & Levine, M. (1996). Reasonable cause: A qualitative study of mandated reporting. *Child Abuse and Neglect, 20,* 275–287.

della Femina, D. D., Yeager, C. A., & Lewis, D. O. (1990). Child abuse: Adolescent records vs. adult recall. *Child Abuse and Neglect, 14,* 227–231.

Department of Health and Human Services, Administration on Children, Youth and Families. (1998). *Child maltreatment 1996: Reports from the states to the National Child Abuse and Neglect Data System.* Washington, DC: U.S. Government Printing Office.

Department of Health and Human Services, Administration on Children, Youth and Families. (1999). *Child maltreatment 1997: Reports from the states to the National Child Abuse and Neglect Data System.* Washington, DC: U.S. Government Printing Office.

DeVoe, E. R., & Faller, K. C. (1999). The characteristics of disclosure among children who may have been sexually abused. *Child Maltreatment, 4,* 217–227.

DiLillo, D., Tremblay, G. C., & Peterson, L. (2000). Linking childhood sexual abuse and abusive parenting: The mediating role of maternal anger. *Child Abuse and Neglect, 24,* 767–780.

Dodge, K. A., Pettit, G. S., Bates, J. E., & Valente, E. (1995). Social information-processing patterns partially mediates the effect of early physical abuse on later conduct problems. *Journal of Abnormal Psychology, 104,* 632–643.

Downing, C. J. (1985). Referrals that work. *School Counselor, 32,* 242–246.

Dryfoos, J. (1994). *Full-service schools: A revolution in health and social services for children, youth, and families.* San Francisco: Jossey-Bass.

Dubowitz, H. (Ed.) (1999). *Neglected children: Research, practice, and policy.* Thousand Oaks, CA: Sage.

Dubowitz, H., Klockner, A., Starr, R. H., Jr., & Black, M. M. (1998). Community and professional definitions of child neglect. *Child Maltreatment, 3,* 235–243.

Dutton, M. A., & Rubinstein, F. L. (1995). Working with people with PTSD: Research implications. In C. R. Figley (Ed.), *Compassion fatigue: Coping with secondary traumatic stress disorder in those who treat the traumatized* (pp. 82–100). New York: Brunner/Mazel.

Dwyer, K., Osher, D., & Warger, C. (1998). *Early warning, timely response: A guide to safe schools.* Washington, DC: U.S. Department of Education.

Eckenrode, J., Laird, M., & Doris, J. (1993). School performance and disciplinary problems among abused and neglected children. *Developmental Psychology, 29,* 53–62.

Eckenrode, J., Rowe, E., Laird, M., & Brathwaite, J. (1995). Mobility as a mediator of the effects of child maltreatment on academic performance. *Child Development, 66,* 1130–1142.

Edleson, J. L. (1999a, October). *Implications for children who witness abuse: Viewing child development as a determinant of health.* Plenary session presented to the International Conference on Children Exposed to Domestic Violence, Vancouver, British Columbia, Canada.

Edleson, J. L. (1999b). Children's witnessing of adult domestic violence. *Journal of Interpersonal Violence, 14,* 839–870.

English, D. J. (1998). The extent and consequences of child maltreatment. In R. E. Behrman (Ed.), *The future of children: Protecting children from abuse and neglect* (pp. 39–53). Los Altos, CA: The Center for the Future of Children, The David and Lucile Packard Foundation.

English, D. J. (1999). Evaluation and risk assessment of child neglect in public child protection services. In H. Dubowitz (Ed.), *Neglected children: Research, practice, and policy* (pp. 191–210). Thousand Oaks, CA: Sage.

Erickson, M. F., & Egeland, B. (1987). A developmental view of the psychological consequences of maltreatment. *School Psychology Review, 16,* 156–168.

Ethier, L. S., Palacio-Quintin, E., & Jourdan-Ionescu, C. (1992). Abuse and neglect: Two distinct forms of maltreatment? *Canada's Mental Health, 40,* 13–19.

Everill, J., & Waller, G. (1995). Disclosure of sexual abuse and psychological adjustment in female undergraduates. *Child Abuse and Neglect, 19,* 93–100.

Everson, M. D., & Boat, B. W. (1989). False allegations of sexual abuse by children and adolescents. *Journal of the American Academy of Child and Adolescent Psychiatry, 28,* 230–235.

Fagan, T., & Wise, P. S. (1994). *School psychology: Past, present, and future.* New York: Longman.

Faller, K. C. (1996). Interviewing children who have been abused: A historical perspective and overview of controversies. *Child Maltreatment, 1,* 83–95.

Famularo, R., Fenton, T., Kincherff, R., Ayoub, C. & Barnum, R. (1994). Maternal and child posttraumatic stress disorder in cases of child maltreatment. *Child Abuse and Neglect, 18,* 27–36.

Feindler, E. L. (1991). Cognitive strategies in anger control interventions for children and adolescents. In P. C. Kendall (Ed.), *Child and adolescent therapy: Cognitive-behavioral procedures* (pp. 66–97). New York: Guilford Press.

Fewster, G., & Bagley, C. (1986). Detection and treatment of child sexual abuse: Mobilising schools. *Journal of Child Care, 2,* vii-xi.

Figley, C. R. (1989). *Helping traumatized families.* San Francisco: Jossey-Bass.

Figley, C. R. (1995a). Compassion fatigue as secondary traumatic stress disorder: An overview. In C. R. Figley (Ed.), *Compassion fatigue: Coping with secondary traumatic stress disorder in those who treat the traumatized* (pp. 1–20). New York: Brunner/Mazel.

Figley, C. R. (1995b). Compassion fatigue: Toward a new understanding of the costs of caring. In B. H. Stamm (Ed.), *Secondary traumatic stress: Self-care issues for clinicians, researchers, and educators* (pp. 3–28). Lutherville, MD: Sidran Press.

Figley, C. R., & Kleber, R. J. (1995). Beyond the "victim": Secondary traumatic stress. In R. J. Kleber, C. R. Figley, & P. R. Berthold (Eds.), *Beyond trauma: Cultural and societal dynamics* (pp. 75–98). New York: Plenum Press.

Finkelhor, D. (1988). The trauma of child sexual abuse: Two models. *Journal of Interpersonal Violence, 2,* 348–366.

Finkelhor, D. (1994). Current information on the scope and nature of child sexual abuse. In R. E. Behrman (Ed.), *The future of children: Sexual abuse of children* (pp. 31–53). Los Altos, CA: The Center for the Future of Children, The David and Lucile Packard Foundation.

Finkelhor, D., Asdigian, N., & Dziuba-Leatherman, J. (1995). The effectiveness of victimization prevention instruction: An evaluation of children's responses to actual threats and assaults. *Child Abuse and Neglect, 19,* 141–153.

Finkelhor, D., & Baron, L. (1986). High-risk children. In D. Finkelhor (Ed.), *A sourcebook on child sexual abuse.* Beverly Hills, CA: Sage.

Finkelhor, D., & Berliner, L. (1995). Research on the treatment of sexually abused children: A review and recommendations. *Journal of the American Academy of Child and Adolescent Psychiatry, 34,* 1408–1423.

Finkelhor, D., & Dziuba-Leatherman, J. (1994). Children as victims of violence: A national survey. *Pediatrics, 94,* 413–420.

Finkelhor, D., & Dziuba-Leatherman, J. (1995). Victimization prevention programs: A national survey of children's exposure and reactions. *Child Abuse and Neglect, 19,* 129–139.

Finkelhor, D., Hotaling, G., Lewis, I. A., & Smith, C. (1990). Sexual abuse in a national survey of adult men and women: Prevalence, characteristics, and risk factors. *Child Abuse and Neglect, 14,* 19–28.

Finkelhor, D., Mitchell, K., & Wolak, J. (2000). Online victimization: A report on the nation's youth. [Online] Available: *http://www.missingkids.com.*

Ford, J. D., Racusin, R., Ellis, C. G., Daviss, W. B., Reiser, J., Fleischer, A., & Thomas, J. (2000). Child maltreatment, other trauma exposure, and posttraumatic symptomatology among children with Oppositional Defiant and Attention Deficit Hyperactivity Disorders. *Child Maltreatment, 5,* 205–217.

Foxhall, K. (2000, July/August). Locking up child abusers is not enough, psychologist tells Congress. *APA Monitor, 31,* 23.

Friedrich, W. N. (1990). *Psychotherapy of sexually abused children and their families.* New York: Norton.

Friedrich, W. N. (1993). Preface. In E. Gil & T. C. Johnson, *Sexualized children: Assessment and treatment of sexualized children and children who molest* (pp. ix–xii). Rockville, MD: Launch Press.

Friedrich, W. N. (1995). *Psychotherapy with sexually abused boys: An integrated approach.* Thousand Oaks, CA: Sage.

Friedrich, W. N. (1996). An integrated model of psychotherapy for abused children. In J. Briere, L. Berliner, J. A. Bulkley, C. Jenny, & T. Reid (Eds.), *The American Professional Society on the Abuse of Children (APSAC) handbook on child maltreatment* (pp. 104–118). Thousand Oaks, CA: Sage.

Fryer, G. E., Kraizer, S. K., & Miyoshi, T. (1987). Measuring children's retention of skills to resist stranger abduction: Use of the simulation technique. *Child Abuse and Neglect, 11,* 181–185.

Garbarino, J. (1987). Children's response to a sexual abuse prevention program: A study of the Spiderman comic. *Child Abuse and Neglect, 11,* 143–148.

Garbarino, J. (1999). *Lost boys: Why our sons turn violent and how we can save them.* New York: Free Press.

Garbarino, J. (2000, March). *Lost boys: Understanding why our sons turn violent and how we can save them.* Address to the National Association of School Psychologists Convention, New Orleans, LA.

Garbarino, J., & Collins, C. C. (1999). Child neglect: The family with a hole in the middle. In H. Dubowitz (Ed.), *Neglected children: Research, practice, and policy* (pp. 1–23). Thousand Oaks, CA: Sage.

Garbarino, J., Guttman, E., & Seeley, J. (1986). *The psychologically battered child.* San Francisco: Jossey-Bass.

Gaudin, J. M., Jr. (1999). Child neglect: Short-term and long-term outcomes. In H. Dubowitz (Ed.), *Neglected children: Research, practice, and policy* (pp. 89–108). Thousand Oaks, CA: Sage.

Gelardo, M. S., & Sanford, E. E. (1987). Child abuse and neglect: A review of the literature. *School Psychology Review, 16,* 137–155.

Gelles, R. J. (1999). Policy issues in child neglect. In H. Dubowitz (Ed.), *Neglected children: Research, practice, and policy* (pp. 278–298). Thousand Oaks, CA: Sage.

Gelles, R. J., & Straus, M. A. (1988). *Intimate violence.* New York: Simon & Schuster.

Gentles, I., & Cassidy, E. (1988). Child sexual abuse prevention programs and their evaluation: Implications for planning and programing. *Journal of Child Care, 3,* 81–93.

Gil, E. (1987). *Children who molest: A guide for parents of young sex offenders.* Walnut Creek, CA: Launch Press.

Gil, E. (1991). *The healing power of play: Working with abused children.* New York: Guilford Press.

Gil, E., & Johnson, T. C. (1993). *Sexualized children: Assessment and treatment of sexualized children and children who molest.* Rockville, MD: Launch Press.

Goodman, G. S., & Rosenberg, M. S. (1987). The child witness to family violence: Clinical and legal considerations. In D. J. Sonkin (Ed.), *Domestic violence on trial: Psychological and legal dimensions of family violence* (pp. 97–126). New York: Springer.

Gorey, K. M., & Leslie, D. R. (1997). The prevalence of child sexual abuse: Integrative review adjustment for potential response and measurement biases. *Child Abuse and Neglect, 21,* 391–398.

Greenberg, M. T., Domitrovich, C., & Bumbarger, B. (1999). *Preventing mental disorders in school-age children: A review of the effectiveness of prevention programs.* Washington, DC: U.S. Department of Health and Human Services, Center for Mental Health Services.

Gross, A. B., & Keller, H. R. (1992). Long-term consequences of childhood physical and psychological maltreatment. *Aggressive Behavior, 18,* 171–185.

Hagans, K. B., & Case, J. (1988). *When your child has been molested: A parent's guide to healing and recovery.* San Francisco: Jossey-Bass.

Haskett, M. E., & Kistner, J. A. (1991). Social interactions and peer perceptions of young physically abused children. *Child Development, 62,* 979–990.

Hazzard, A., Webb, C., Kleemeier, C., Angert, L., & Pohl, J. (1991). Child sexual abuse prevention: Evaluation and one-year follow-up. *Child Abuse and Neglect, 15,* 123–138.

Helfer, R. E. (1987). The litany of the smoldering neglect of children. In R. E. Helfer & C. H. Kempe (Eds.), *The battered child* (pp. 301–311). Chicago: University of Chicago Press.

Herman, J. L. (1992). *Trauma and recovery.* New York: HarperCollins.

Hindman, J. (1991). *When mourning breaks.* Ontario, OR: AlexAndria Associates.

Hindman, J. (1999). *Just before dawn: From the shadows of tradition to new reflections in trauma assessment and treatment of sexual victimization.* Ontario, OR: AlexAndria Associates.

Holden, E. W., & Nabors, L. (1999). The prevention of child neglect. In H. Dubowitz (Ed.), *Neglected children: Research, practice, and policy* (pp. 174–190). Thousand Oaks, CA: Sage.

Holmes, W. C., & Slap, G. B. (1998). Sexual abuse of boys: Definition, prevalence, correlates, sequelae, and management. *Journal of the American Medical Association, 280,* 1855–1862.

Horton, C. B. (1995). Best practices in the response to child maltreatment. In A. Thomas & T. Grimes (Eds.), *Best practices in school psychology—III* (pp. 963–976). Silver Spring, MD: National Association of School Psychologists.

Horton, C. B. (1996). Children who molest other children: The school psychologist's response to the sexually aggressive child. *School Psychology Review, 25,* 540–557.

Horton, C. B., & Cruise, T. K. (1997a). Child sexual abuse. In G. G. Bear, K. M. Minke, & A. Thomas (Eds.), *Children's needs: II. Development, problems and alternatives* (pp. 719–727). Bethesda, MD: National Association of School Psychologists.

Horton, C. B., & Cruise, T. K. (1997b). Clinical assessment of child victims and adult survivors of child maltreatment. *Journal of Counseling and Development, 76,* 94–104.

Horton, C. B., Cruise, T. K., Graybill, D., & Cornett, J. Y. (1999). For children's sake: Training students in the treatment of child witnesses of domestic violence. *Professional Psychology: Research and Practice, 30,* 88–91.

Horton, C. B., & Oakland, T. (1996). *Classroom applications of the SSQ.* San Antonio, TX: Psychological Corporation.

House, A. E. (1999). *DSM-IV diagnosis in the schools.* New York: Guilford Press.

Huebner, E. S. (1992). Burnout among school psychologists: An exploratory investigation into its nature, extent, and correlates. *School Psychology Quarterly, 7,* 129–136.

Huebner, E. S. (1993). Burnout among school psychologists in the USA: Further data related to its prevalence and correlates. *School Psychology International, 14,* 99–109.

Huebner, E. S. (1994). Relationships among demographics, social support, job satisfaction and burnout among school psychologists. *School Psychology International, 15,* 181–186.

Illinois Department of Child and Family Services. (1998). *A manual for mandated reporter.s* Springfield, IL: Author.

Jaffe, P. G., Sudermann, M., & Reitzel, D. (1992). Child witnesses of marital violence. In R. T. Ammerman & M. Hersen (Eds.), *Assessment of family violence: A clinical and legal sourcebook* (pp. 313–331). New York: Wiley.

Jaffe, P. G., Wolfe, D. A., & Wilson, S. K. (1990). *Children of battered women.* Newbury Park, CA: Sage.

James, S. H., & Burch, K. M. (1999). School counselors' roles in cases of child sexual behavior. *Professional School Counseling, 2,* 211–217.

Johnson, T. C. (1989). Female child perpetrators: Children who molest other children. *Child Abuse and Neglect, 13,* 571–585.

Johnson, T. C. (1990). Children who act out sexually. In J. McNamara & B. H. McNamara (Eds.), *Adoption and the sexually abused child* (pp. 63–73). Portland, ME: Human Services Development Institute, University of Southern Maine.

Johnson, T. C. (1995). *Treatment exercises for child abuse victims and children with sexual behavior problems.* Pasadena, CA: Author.

Johnson, T. C. (1999). *Understanding your child's sexual behavior: What's natural and healthy.* Oakland, CA: New Harbinger.

Johnson, T. C., & Friend, C. (1995). Assessing young children's sexual behaviors in the context of child sexual abuse evaluations. In T. Ney (Ed.), *True and false allegations of child sexual abuse: Assessment and case management* (pp. 49–72). New York: Brunner/Mazel.

Jones, D. P., & McGraw, J. M. (1987). Reliable and fictitious accounts of sexual abuse to children. *Journal of Interpersonal Violence, 2,* 27–45.

Kahn, T. J. (1996). *Pathways: A guided workbook for youth beginning treatment.* Brandon, VT: Safer Society Press.

Kahn, T. (1999). *Roadmaps to recovery: A guided workbook for young people in treatment.* Brandon, VT: Safer Society Press.

Kaplan, S. J., Pelcovitz, D., & Labruna, V. (1999). Child and adolescent abuse and neglect research: A review of the past 10 years. Part I: Physical and emotional abuse and neglect. *Journal of the American Academy of Child and Adolescent Psychiatry, 38,* 1214–1222.

Karen, R. (1994). *Becoming attached: First relationships and how they shape our capacity to love.* New York: Oxford University Press.

Kassam-Adams, N. (1995). The risks of treating sexual trauma: Stress and secondary trauma in psychotherapists. In B. H. Stamm (Ed.), *Secondary traumatic stress: Self-care issues for clinicians, researchers, and educators* (pp. 37–48). Lutherville, MD: Sidran Press.

Kaufman, J., & Cicchetti, D. (1989). Effects of maltreatment on school-age children's socioemotional development: Assessments in a day-camp setting. *Developmental Psychology, 25,* 516–524.

Kaufman, K. L., Holmberg, J. K., Orts, K. A., McCrady, F. E., Rotzien, A. L., Daleiden, E. L., & Hilliker, D. R. (1998). Factors influencing sexual offenders' modus operandi: An examination of victim–offender relatedness and age. *Child Maltreatment, 3* (4), 349–361.

Kegan, R. (1982). *The evolving self.* Cambridge, MA: Harvard University Press.

Kempe, C. H., & Helfer, R. (Eds.). (1980). *The battered child* (3rd ed.). Chicago: University of Chicago Press.

Kendall, P. C. (Ed.). (1991). *Child and adolescent therapy: Cognitive-behavioral procedures.* New York: Guilford Press.

Kendall, P. C., Chansky, T. E., Freidman, M., Kim, R., Kortlander, E., Sessa, F. M., & Siqueland, L. (1991). Treating anxiety disorders in children and adolescents. In P. C. Kendall (Ed.), *Child and adolescent therapy: Cognitive-behavioral procedures* (pp. 131–164). New York: Guilford Press.

Kendall-Tackett, K. A. (2000). Physiological correlates of childhood abuse: Chronic hyperarousal in PTSD, depression, and irritable bowel syndrome. *Child Abuse and Neglect, 24,* 799–810.

Kendall-Tackett, K. A., Williams, L. M., & Finkelhor, D. (1993). Impact of sexual abuse on children: A review and synthesis of recent empirical studies. *Psychological Bulletin, 113,* 164–180.

Kikuchi, J. J. (1995). When the offender is a child: Identifying and responding to juvenile sexual abuse offenders. In M. Hunter (Ed.), *Child survivors and perpetrators of sexual abuse: Treatment innovations* (pp. 108–124). Thousand Oaks, CA: Sage.

Kolko, D. J. (1992). Characteristics of child victims of physical violence: Research findings and clinical implications. *Journal of Interpersonal Violence, 7,* 244–276.

Kolko, D. J. (1996a). Child physical abuse. In J. Briere, L. Berliner, J. A. Bulkley, C. Jenny, & T. Reid (Eds.), *The American Professional Society on the Abuse of Children (APSAC) handbook on child maltreatment* (pp. 21–50). Thousand Oaks, CA: Sage.

Kolko, D. J. (1996b). Individual cognitive behavioral therapy and family therapy for physically abused children and their offending parents: A comparison of clinical outcomes. *Child Maltreatment, 1,* 322–342.

Koralek, D. G. (1992). *Caregivers of young children: Preventing and responding to child maltreatment.* Washington, DC: National Clearinghouse on Child Abuse and Neglect Information.

Krugman, R., & Jones, D. P. H. (1987). Incest and other forms of sexual abuse. In R. E. Helfer & R. E. Kempe (Eds.), *The battered child* (pp. 286–300). Chicago: University of Chicago Press.

Kurtz, P. D., Gaudin, J. M., Jr., Wodarski, J. S., & Howing, P. T. (1993). Maltreatment and the school-aged child: School performance consequences. *Child Abuse and Neglect, 17,* 581–589.

Lamb, M. E. (1994). The investigation of child sexual abuse: An interdisciplinary consensus statement. *Journal of Child Sexual Abuse, 3,* 93–106.

Larson, C., Terman, D., Gomby, D., Quinn, L., & Behrman, R. (1994). Sexual abuse of children: Recommendations and analysis. In R. E. Behrman (Ed.), *The future of children: Sexual abuse of children* (pp. 4–30). Los Altos, CA: The Center for the Future of Children, The David and Lucile Packard Foundation.

Lee, I., & Sylvester, K. (1997). *When mommy got hurt: A story for young children about domestic violence.* Indianapolis: Kidsrights.

Leiter, J., & Johnsen, M. C. (1997). Child maltreatment and school performance declines: An event-history analysis. *American Educational Research Journal, 34,* 563–589.

Levine, M., Doueck, H. J., Anderson, E. M., Chavez, F. T., Deisz, R. L., George, N. A., Sharma, A., Steinberg, K. L., & Wallach, L. (1995). *The impact of mandated reporting on the therapeutic relationship: Picking up the pieces.* Thousand Oaks, CA: Sage.

Lewis, D. O. (1992). From abuse to violence: Psychophysiological consequences of maltreatment. *Journal of the American Academy of Child and Adolescent Psychiatry, 31,* 383–391.

Lindon, J., & Nourse, C. A. (1994). A multi-dimensional model of groupwork for adolescent girls who have been sexually abused. *Child Abuse and Neglect, 18,* 341–348.

Linehan, M. M. (1993). *Skills training manual for treating borderline personality disorder.* New York: Guilford Press.

Lochman, J. E., White, K. J., & Wayland, K. K. (1991). Cognitive-behavioral assessment and treatment with aggressive children. In P. C. Kendall (Ed.), *Child and adolescent therapy: Cognitive-behavioral procedures* (pp. 25–65). New York: Guilford Press.

Loftus, E. F., & Yapko, M. D. (1995). In T. Ney (Ed.), *True and false allegations of child sexual abuse: Assessment and case management* (pp. 176–191). New York: Brunner/Mazel.

Longo, R. E., & Groth, A. N. (1983). Juvenile sexual offenses in the histories of adult rapists and child molesters. *International Journal of Offender Therapy and Comparative Criminology, 27,* 150–155.

Lorber, R., Felton, D. K., & Reid, J. B. (1985). A social learning approach to the reduction of coercive processes in child abusive families: A molecular analysis. *Advances in Behaviour Research and Therapy, 6,* 29–45.

Lyon, T. D. (1999). Are battered women bad mothers? Rethinking the termination of abused women's parental rights for failure to protect. In H. Dubowitz (Ed.), *Neglected children: Research, practice, and policy* (pp. 237–260). Thousand Oaks, CA: Sage.

Maital, S. L. (1996). Integration of behavioral and mental health consultation as a means of overcoming resistance. *Journal of Educational and Psychological Consultation, 7,* 291–304.

Maker, A. H., Kemmelmeier, M., & Peterson, C. (1998). Long-term psychological consequences in women of witnessing parental physical conflict and experiencing abuse in childhood. *Journal of Interpersonal Violence, 13,* 574–589.

Margolin, G. (1998). Effects of domestic violence on children. In P. K. Trickett & C. J. Schellenbach (Eds.), *Violence against children in the family and the community* (pp. 57–101). Washington, DC: American Psychological Association.

Marion, M. (1982). Primary prevention of child abuse: The role of the family life educator. *Family Relations, 31,* 575–582.

Mather, C. L., Debye, K. E., & Wood, J. (1994). *How long does it hurt?: A guide to recovering from incest and sexual abuse for teenagers, their friends, and their families.* San Francisco: Jossey-Bass.

Mayhall, P. D., & Norgard, K. E. (1983). *Child abuse and neglect: Sharing responsibility.* New York: Wiley.

McCloskey, L. A., Figueredo, A. J., & Koss, M. P. (1995). The effects of systematic family violence on children's mental health. *Child Development, 66,* 1239–1261.

Meichenbaum, D. (1997). *Treating post-traumatic stress disorder: A handbook and practice manual for therapy.* Brisbane, Australia: Wiley.

Milgram, J. (1984). Physical and sexual child abuse: Implications for middle level professionals. *NASSP Bulletin, 68,* 58–62.

Miller-Perrin, C. L., & Perrin, R. D. (1999). *Child maltreatment: An introduction.* Thousand Oaks, CA: Sage.

Mills, L. B., & Huebner, E. S. (1998). A prospective study of personality characteristics, occupational stressors, and burnout among school psychology practitioners. *Journal of School Psychology, 36,* 103–120.

Milner, J. S. (1998). Individual and family characteristics associated with intrafamilial child physical and sexual abuse. In P. K. Trickett & C. J. Schellenbach (Eds.), *Violence against children in the family and the community* (pp. 141–170). Washington, DC: American Psychological Association.

Morgan, S. R. (1994). Child abuse and neglect. In S. R. Morgan (Ed.), *At-risk youth in crises: A team approach in the schools* (pp. 117–178). Austin, TX: Pro-ed.

Mullen, P. E., Martin, J. L., Anderson, J. C., Romans, S. E., & Herbison, G. P. (1996). The long-term impact of the physical, emotional, and sexual abuse of children: A community study. *Child Abuse and Neglect, 20,* 7–21.

Munroe, J. F. (1995). Ethical issues associated with secondary trauma in therapists. In B. H. Stamm (Ed.), *Secondary traumatic stress: Self-care issues for clinicians, researchers, and educators* (pp. 211–229). Lutherville, MD: Sidran Press.

National Center on Child Abuse and Neglect. (1988). *Study findings: Study of national incidence and prevalence of child abuse and neglect* (DHHS Publication No. 105–85–1702). Washington, DC: U.S. Government Printing Office.

National Clearinghouse on Child Abuse and Neglect Information. (2000, January 19). *Prevention Fundamentals* [Online]. Available: *http://www.calib.com/nccanch/prevmnth/programs/fundamentals.htm.*

Newman, M. R., & Lutzker, J. R. (1990). Prevention programs. In R. T. Ammerman & M. Hersen (Eds.), *Children at-risk: An evaluation of factors contributing to child abuse and neglect.* New York: Plenum Press.

Nugent, M., Labram, A., & McLoughlin, L. (1998). The effects of child sexual abuse on school life. *Educational and Child Psychology, 15,* 68–78.

O'Donohue, W., Geer, J. H., & Elliott, A. (1992). The primary prevention of child sexual abuse. In W. O'Donohue & J. H. Geer (Eds.), *The sexual abuse of children: Clinical issues* (Vol. 2, pp. 477–517). Hillsdale, NJ: Erlbaum.

O'Donohue, W., & O'Hare, E. (1997). How do teachers react to children labeled as sexually abused? *Child Maltreatment, 2,* 46–51.

O'Donohue, W., & Rudman, J. C. (1999). Social relations of sexually abused children: A social information processing analysis. *Aggression and Violent Behavior, 4,* 29–39.

Osofsky, J. D., & Scheeringa, M. S. (1997). Community and domestic violence exposure: Effects on development and psychopathology. In D. Cicchetti & S. L. Toth (Eds.), *Developmental perspectives on trauma: Theory, research, and intervention* (pp. 155–180). Rochester, NY: University of Rochester Press.

O'Toole, R., Webster, S. W., O'Toole, A. W., & Lucal, B. (1999). Teacher's recognition and reporting of child abuse: A factorial survey. *Child Abuse and Neglect, 23,* 1083–1101.

Pearlman, L. A. (1995). Self-care for trauma therapists: Ameliorating vicarious traumatization. In B. H. Stamm (Ed.), *Secondary traumatic stress: Self-care issues for clinicians, researchers, and educators* (pp. 51–64). Lutherville, MD: Sidran Press.

Pearlman, L. A., & Mac Ian, P. S. (1995). Vicarious traumatization: An empirical study of the effects of trauma work on trauma therapists. *Professional Psychology: Research and Practice, 26,* 558–565.

Pelzer, D. (1995). *A child called "It": One child's courage to survive.* Deerfield Beach, FL: Health Communications.

Peters, S. D., Wyatt, G. E., & Finkelhor, D. (1986). Prevalence. In D. Finkelhor (Ed.), *Sourcebook on child sexual abuse* (pp. 15–59). Newbury Park, CA: Sage.

Peterson, M. S., & Urquiza, A. J. (1993). *The role of mental health professionals in the prevention and treatment of child abuse and neglect.* Washington, DC: U.S. Department of Health and Human Services, Administration on Children, Youth and Families.

Pezdek, K., & Hodge, D. (1999). Planting false childhood memories in children: The role of event plausibility. *Child Development, 70,* 887–895.

Polansky, N. A., & Williams, D. P. (1978). Class orientations to child neglect. *Social Work, 23,* 397–401.

Pope, K. F., & Vasquez, M. J. T. (1991). *Ethics in psychotherapy and counseling.* San Francisco: Jossey-Bass.

Price, J. M., & Landsverk, J. (1998). Social information-processing patterns as predictors of social adaptation and behavior problems among maltreated children in foster care. *Child Abuse and Neglect, 22,* 845–858.

Reed, L. D. (1994). A commentary on content and process of the interdisciplinary consensus statement. *Journal of Child Sexual Abuse, 3,* 123–127.

Reed, L. D. (1996). Findings from research on children's suggestibility and implications for conducting child interviews. *Child Maltreatment, 1,* 105–120.

Reiniger, A., Robison, E., & McHugh, M. (1995). Mandated training of professionals: A means for improving reporting of suspected child abuse. *Child Abuse and Neglect, 19,* 63–69.

Rind, B., Tromovitch, P., & Bauserman, R. (1998). A meta-analytic examination of assumed properties of child sexual abuse using college samples. *Psychological Bulletin, 124,* 22–53.

Rispens, J., Aleman, A., & Goudena, P. P. (1997). Prevention of child sexual abuse victimization: A meta-analysis of school programs. *Child Abuse and Neglect, 21,* 975–987.

Roesler, T. A. (1994) Reactions to disclosure of child sexual abuse: The effect on adult symptoms. *Journal of Nervous and Mental Disease, 182,* 618–624.

Rosenbaum, A., & O'Leary, K. D. (1981). Children: The unintended victims of marital violence. *American Journal of Orthopsychiatry, 51,* 692–699.

Ryan, G. (1989). Victim to victimizer: Re-thinking victim treatment. *Journal of Interpersonal Violence, 4,* 325–341.

Ryan, G. (1997). Sexually abusive youth: Defining the population. In G. Ryan & S. Lane (Eds.), *Juvenile sex offending: Causes, consequences, and correction* (pp. 3–18). San Francisco: Jossey-Bass.

Ryan, G., & Lane, S. (Eds.). (1997a). *Juvenile sexual offending: Causes, consequences, and correction.* San Francisco: Jossey-Bass.

Ryan, G., & Lane, S. (1997b). The impact of sexual abuse on the interventionist. In G. Ryan & S. Lane (Eds.), *Juvenile sexual offending: Causes, consequences, and correction* (pp. 457–474). San Francisco: Jossey-Bass.

Saakvitne, K. W., & Pearlman, L. A. (1996). *Transforming the pain: A workbook on vicarious traumatization.* New York: Norton.

Salter, A. C. (1988). *Treating child sex offenders and victims: A practical guide.* Newbury Park, CA: Sage.

Salzinger, S. (1999). Determinants of abuse and the effects of violence on children and adolescents. In A. J. Goreczny & M. Hersen (Eds.), *Handbook of pediatric and adolescent health psychology* (pp. 429–449). Boston: Allyn & Bacon.

Sarno, J. A., & Wurtele, S. K. (1997). Effects of a personal safety program on preschoolers' knowledge, skills, and perceptions of child sexual abuse. *Child Maltreatment, 2,* 35–45.

Satullo, J., & Bradway, R. (1987). *It happens to boys too.* Pittsfield, MA: Elizabeth Freeman Center.

Saunders, B. E., & Williams, L. M. (1996). Introduction to special section regarding treatment outcome studies. *Child Maltreatment, 1,* 293.

Saywitz, K. J., & Goodman, G. S. (1996). Interviewing children in and out of court: Current research and practice implications. In J. Briere, L. Berliner, J. A. Bulkley, C. Jenny, & T. Reid (Eds.), *The American Professional Society on the Abuse of Children* (APSAC) handbook on child maltreatment (pp. 297–318). Thousand Oaks, CA: Sage.

Schaaf, K. K., & McCanne, T. R. (1998). Relationship of childhood sexual, physical, and combined sexual and physical abuse to adult victimization and posttraumatic stress disorder. *Child Abuse and Neglect, 22,* 1119–1133.

Schauben, L. J., & Frazier, P. A. (1995). Vicarious trauma: The effects on female counselors of working with sexual violence survivors. *Psychology of Women Quarterly, 19,* 49–64.

Sedlack, A. J., & Broadhurst, D. D. (1996). *Third national incidence study on child abuse and neglect.* Washington, DC: U.S. Department of Health and Human Services.

Seligman, M. E. P. (1975). *Helplessness: On depression, development and death.* San Francisco: W. H. Freeman.

Seryak, J. M. (1997). *Dear teacher, if you only knew . . . : Adults recovering from child sexual abuse speak to educators.* Bath, OH: The Dear Teacher Project.

Shoop, R. J., & Firestone, L. M. (1988). Mandatory reporting of suspected child abuse: Do teachers obey the law? *West's Education Law Reporter, 46,* 1115–1122.

Skinner, C. H. (1999). Prevention and remediation through group intervention. *School Psychology Quarterly, 14,* 189–194.

Slater, B. R., & Gallagher, M. M. (1989). Outside the realm of psychotherapy: Consultation for interventions with sexualized children. *School Psychology Review, 18,* 400–411.

Sorenson, T., & Snow, B. (1991). How children tell: The process of disclosure in sexual abuse. *Child Welfare, 70,* 3–15.

Stahley, G., & Adamson, J. (1999, October). *Custody and access in domestic violence cases: Clinical issues, legal trends, research findings and recommendations.* Paper presented to the International Conference on Children Exposed to Domestic Violence, Vancouver, British Columbia, Canada.

Stark, K., Rouse, L. W., & Livingston, R. (1991). Treatment of depression during childhood and adolescence: Cognitive-behavioral procedures. In P. C. Kendall (Ed.), *Child and adolescent therapy: Cognitive-behavioral procedures* (pp. 165–206). New York: Guilford Press.

Steen, C. (1997). *The relapse prevention book for youth in treatment.* Brandon, VT: Safer Society Press.

Straus, M. A. (1992). Sociological research and social policy: The case of family violence. *Sociological Forum, 7,* 211–237.

Sudermann, M., Jaffe, P. G., & Hastings, E. (1995). Violence prevention programs in secondary (high) schools. In E. Peled, P. G. Jaffe, & J. L. Edleson (Eds.), *Ending the cycle of violence: Community responses to children of battered women* (pp. 232–254). Thousand Oaks, CA: Sage.

Terr, L. C. (1991). Childhood traumas: An outline and overview. *American Journal of Psychiatry, 148,* 10–20.

Tharinger, D. (1987). Children and sexual interest. In A. Thomas & J. Grimes (Eds.), *Children's needs: Psychological perspectives* (pp. 532–542). Kent, OH: National Association of School Psychologists.

Tharinger, D. (1991, August). Recovery from child sexual abuse: Research findings and implications for school psychologists. In D. Tharinger (Chair), *School psychologists' response to child abuse: Training, practice, and research.* Symposium conducted at the annual convention of the American Psychological Association, San Francisco, CA.

Tharinger, D., & Horton, C. B. (1992). Family–school partnerships: The response to child sexual abuse as a challenging example. In S. L. Christenson & J. C. Conoley (Eds.), *Home school collaboration: Enhancing children's academic and social competence* (pp. 467–486). Silver Spring, MD: National Association of School Psychologists.

Tharinger, D. J., Krivacska, J. J., Laye-McDonough, M., Jamison, L., Vincent, G. G., & Hedlund, A. D. (1988). Prevention of child sexual abuse: An analysis of issues, educational programs, and research findings. *School Psychology Review, 17,* 614–634.

Tharinger, D., Russian, T., & Robinson, P. (1989). School psychologists' involvement in the response to child sexual abuse. *School Psychology Review, 18,* 386–399.

Tharinger, D., & Vevier, E. (1987). Child sexual abuse: A review and intervention framework for the teacher. *Journal of Research and Development in Education, 20,* 12–24.

Tite, R. (1994). Detecting the symptoms of child abuse: Classroom complications. *Canadian Journal of Education, 19,* 1–14.

Tomison, A. M., & Tucci, J. (1997). Emotional abuse: The hidden form of maltreatment. *Issues in Child Abuse Prevention, 8,* 1–30.

Tower, C. C. (1987). *How schools can help combat child abuse and neglect.* Washington, DC: National Education Association.

Tower, C. C. (1992). *The role of educators in the prevention and treatment of child abuse and neglect.* Washington, DC: U.S. Department of Health and Human Services, Administration on Children, Youth and Families.

Tutty, L. M. (1994). Developmental issues in young children's learning of sexual abuse prevention concepts. *Child Abuse and Neglect, 18,* 179–192.

van der Kolk, B. A. (1989). The compulsion to repeat the trauma: Re-enactment, revictimization, and masochism. *Psychiatric Clinics of North America, 12,* 389–411.

Verduyn, C., & Calam, R. (1999). Cognitive behavioral interventions with maltreated children and adolescents. *Child Abuse and Neglect, 23,* 197–207.

Vevier, E., & Tharinger, D. J. (1986). Child sexual abuse: A review and intervention framework for the school psychologist. *Journal of School Psychology, 24,* 293–311.

Vissing, Y. M., Straus, M. A., Gelles, R. J., & Harrop, J. W. (1991). Verbal aggression by parents and psychosocial problems of children. *Child Abuse and Neglect, 15,* 223–238.

Volpe, R. (1980). Schools and the problem of child abuse: An introduction and overview. In R. Volpe, M. Breton, & J. Mitton (Eds.), *The maltreatment of the school-aged child* (pp. 3–10). Lexington, MA: Lexington Books.

Wade, P., & Bernstein, B. L. (1991). Culture sensitivity training and counselor's race:

Effects on Black female clients' perceptions and attrition. *Journal of Counseling Psychology, 38,* 9–15.

Walker, E. A., Keegan, D., Gardner, G., Sullivan, M., Bernstein, D., & Katon, W. J. (1997). Psychosocial factors in fibromyalgia compared with rheumatoid arthritis: II. Sexual, physical, and emotional abuse and neglect. *Psychosomatic Medicine, 59,* 572–577.

Wang, C. T., & Daro, D. (1998). *Current trends in child abuse reporting and fatalities: The results of the 1997 annual fifty state survey.* Chicago: National Center on Child Abuse Prevention Research.

Wasserman, R. (1998). *Feeling good again: A workbook for children 6 and up who have been sexually abused.* Brandon, VT: Safer Society Press.

Webersinn, A. L., Hollinger, C. L., & DeLamatre, J. E. (1991). Breaking the cycle of violence: An examination of factors relevant to treatment follow-through. *Psychological Reports, 68,* 231–240.

Wheeler, J. R., & Berliner, L. (1988). Treating the effects of sexual abuse on children. In G. E. Wyatt & G. Powell (Eds.), *Lasting effects of child sexual abuse* (pp. 227–247). Newbury Park: Sage.

Williams, L. M. (1994). Recall of childhood trauma: A prospective study of women's memories of child sexual abuse. *Journal of Consulting and Clinical Psychology, 62,* 1167–1176.

Wilson, C. A., & Gettinger, M. (1989). Determinants of child-abuse reporting among Wisconsin school psychologists. *Professional School Psychology, 4,* 91–102.

Wind, T. W., & Silvern, L. E. (1992). Type and extent of child abuse as predictors of adult functioning. *Journal of Family Violence, 7,* 261–281.

Wolfe, D. A., & Jaffe, P. G. (1999). Emerging strategies in the prevention of domestic violence. In R. E. Behrman (Ed.), *The future of children: Domestic violence and children* (pp. 133–144). Los Altos, CA: The Center for the Future of Children, The David and Lucile Packard Foundation.

Wolfe, D. A., Sas, L., & Wekerle, C. (1994). Factors associated with the development of posttraumatic stress disorder among child victims of sexual abuse. *Child Abuse and Neglect, 18,* 37–50.

Wolfe, D. A., Wekerle, C., Reitzel-Jaffe, D., & Lefebvre, L. (1998). Factors associated with abusive relationships among maltreated and nonmaltreated youth. *Development and Psychopathology, 10,* 61–85.

Wurtele, S. K. (1998). School-based child sexual abuse prevention programs: Questions, answers, and more questions. In J. R. Lutzker (Ed.), *Handbook of child abuse research and treatment* (pp. 501–516). New York: Plenum Press.

Wurtele, S. K., Marrs, S. R., & Miller-Perrin, C. L. (1987). Practice makes perfect? The role of participant modeling in sexual abuse prevention programs. *Journal of Consulting and Clinical Psychology, 55,* 599–602.

Wyncoop, T. F., Capps, S. C., & Priest, B. J. (1995). Incidence and prevalence of child sexual abuse: A critical review of data collection procedures. *Journal of Child Sexual Abuse, 4,* 49–66.

Youngblade, L. M., & Belsky, J. (1990). Social and emotional consequences of child maltreatment. In R. T. Ammerman & M. Hersen (Eds.), *Children at-risk: An evaluation of factors contributing to child abuse and neglect* (pp. 107–146). New York: Plenum Press.

Yuille, J. C., Tymofievich, M., & Marxsen, D. (1995). The nature of allegations of child sexual abuse. In T. Ney (Ed.), *True and false allegations of child sexual abuse: Assessment and case management* (pp. 21–46). New York: Brunner/Mazel.

Zellman, G. L. (1990). Linking schools and social services: The case of child abuse reporting. *Educational Evaluation and Policy Analysis, 12,* 41–55.

Zellman, G., & Faller, K. C. (1996). Reporting of child maltreatment. In J. Briere, L. Berliner, J. A., Bulkley, C. Jenny, & T. Reid (Eds.), *The American Professional Society on the Abuse of Children (APSAC) handbook on child maltreatment* (pp. 359–381). Thousand Oaks, CA: Sage.

◆◆◆
Index
◆